PHARMACY

PHARMACY

EXAMINATION REVIEW

NINTH EDITION

1500 MULTIPLE CHOICE QUESTIONS AND EXPLANATORY ANSWERS

Robert J. Gerraughty, Ph.D.
Vice President for Administration
Creighton University
Omaha, Nebraska

Contributing Editor
Frank Palmiere, R.P.H.
Westchester County Medical Center
New York

CBS

CBS Publishers & Distributors Pvt. Ltd.

New Delhi • Bengaluru • Chennai • Kochi • Kolkata • Mumbai
Hyderabad • Nagpur • Patna • Pune • Vijayawada

ISBN: 81-239-1286-2

First Indian Edition: 1998
Reprint: 2000

Reprinted in India by CBS Publishers & Distributors in arrangement with Elsevier Science Publishing Company, Inc.

Published by **Satish Kumar Jain** and produced by **Varun Jain** for
CBS Publishers & Distributors Pvt. Ltd.,
4819/XI Prahlad Street, 24 Ansari Road, Daryaganj, New Delhi - 110002
delhi@cbspd.com, cbspubs@airtelmail.in • www.cbspd.com
Ph.: 23289259, 23266861, 23266867 • Fax: 011-23243014

Corporate Office: 204 FIE, Industrial Area, Patparganj, Delhi - 110 092
Ph: 49344934 • Fax: 011-49344935
E-mail: publishing@cbspd.com • publicity@cbspd.com

Branches:
- ***Bengaluru:*** 2975, 17th Cross, K.R. Road, Bansankari 2nd Stage, Bengaluru - 70 • Ph: +91-80-26771678/79 • Fax: +91-80-26771680 E-mail: cbsbng@gmail.com, bangalore@cbspd.com
- ***Chennai:*** No. 7, Subbaraya Street, Shenoy Nagar, Chennai - 600030 Ph: +91-44-26681266, 26680620 • Fax: +91-44-42032115 E-mail: chennai@cbspd.com
- ***Kochi:*** Ashana House, 39/1904, A.M. Thomas Road, Valanjambalam, Ernakulum, Kochi • Ph: +91-484-4059061-65 Fax: +91-484-4059065 • E-mail: cochin@cbspd.com
- ***Kolkata:*** 6-B, Ground Floor, Rameshwar Shaw Road, Kolkata - 700014 Ph: +91-33-22891126/7/8 • E-mail: kolkata@cbspd.com
- ***Mumbai:*** 83-C, Dr. E. Moses Road, Worli, Mumbai - 400018 Ph: +91-9833017933, 022-24902340/41 • E-mail: mumbai@cbspd.com

Representatives:
- Hyderabad: 0-9885175004
- Nagpur: 0-9021734563
- Patna: 0-9334159340
- Pune: 0-9623451994
- Vijayawada: 0-9000660880

Printed at:
Neekunj Print Process, Delhi (India)

Contents

Preface

The purpose of this text is to provide an opportunity to determine one's ability to comprehend and apply the vast accumulation of knowledge in this field. It is designed to enable the reader to detect specific areas of strength and weakness in his or her understanding of the subject matter. To further aid in achieving this goal, this text features the inclusion of fully detailed explanatory answers. The discussions of the answers are provided to clarify the selection of answers, to encourage further development in specific problem areas, to test the reader's memory and understanding of basic, factual information, to relate latest concepts and advances in various topics, and to determine problem-solving ability and increase the reader's awareness of underlying principles through the application of factual knowledge to practical situations.

The variations in test questions are offered for increased familiarization with the different types of national, state, and school examinations in use today, and as an opportunity for improving one's skills with multiple choice examinations.

1. PHARMACY

DIRECTIONS: For each of the following multiple choice and matching questions, choose the one most appropriate answer.

---

1. Which of the following is used to prevent dehydration or achieve rehydration?
   A. Lytren solution
   B. Liposul
   C. Bicytra
   D. Mylicon
   E. Simethicone

2. Emulsions made with tweens are usually
   A. unstable
   B. w/o
   C. o/w
   D. clear
   E. reversible

3. Amorphous forms of drugs are
   A. usually less soluble than crystal forms
   B. usually more soluble than crystal forms
   C. also called solvates
   D. practically insoluble
   E. usually less active than other metastable polymorphs

4. A roller mill is used mainly to reduce particle size in
   A. tablet granulations
   B. ointments
   C. capsules
   D. bulk powders
   E. emulsions

5. Particle size reduction will NOT enhance the absorption of
   A. hydrophobic compounds
   B. hydrophilic compounds
   C. weak acids
   D. weak bases
   E. none of the above

6. A liquid whose viscosity is increased when stress is applied is classed as which of the following materials?
   A. Dilatant
   B. Newtonian
   C. Plastic
   D. Pseudoplastic
   E. Thixotrophic

7. A solution contains 3 gr of a drug per fluid ounce. What is the % w/v of the solution?
   A. 0.66%
   B. 0.59%
   C. 10%
   D. 1.0%
   E. 6.5%

8. Cyanocobalamin is a(an)
   A. steroid
   B. choline esterase inhibitor
   C. hallucinogen
   D. vitamin
   E. enzyme

9. Spans and tweens are
   A. highly polymerized mannuronic acid anhydrides
   B. phospholipids
   C. polyoxyalkalene derivatives
   D. glycosides
   E. none of the above

10. Which of the following is NOT a method of splitting emulsions?
   A. Centrifuging
   B. Filtering
   C. Addition of electrolytes
   D. Heat
   E. Addition of a liquid in which both phases are soluble

11. Iron preparations may stain the urine
   A. red
   B. black
   C. orange
   D. purple
   E. brown

12. Lidocaine HCl is not administered orally because it is
   A. ineffective by this route
   B. too acidic
   C. too toxic by this route
   D. a cause of arrhythmias
   E. unstable

13. When phenol is oxidized, its color is
   A. black
   B. pink
   C. brown
   D. yellow
   E. white

14. In preparing a pint of a 1:5000 solution of $HgCl_2$, a pharmacist should use
   A. 190 mg
   B. 95 mg
   C. 19 mg
   D. 9.5 mg
   E. none of the above

15. Which of the following interacts with vasopressin?
   A. Chloramphenicol
   B. Diphenylhydantoin
   C. Chlorpropamide
   D. Dicumarol
   E. Phenprocoumon

16. The two major properties of drugs that are usually modified by complexation are
    A. odor and taste
    B. taste and solubility
    C. chemical structure and solubility
    D. chemical structure and stability
    E. stability and solubility

17. What will result if the distribution of drugs is slower than the processes of biotransformation and elimination?
    A. High blood levels of drug
    B. Low blood levels of drug
    C. Synergism
    D. Potentiation
    E. Failure to attain diffusion equilibrium

18 The term PSIG is reference to aerosols means
    A. propellant safety in glass
    B. per square inch of glass
    C. pounds per square inch gauge
    D. atmospheric pressure
    E. none of the above

19. In radiopharmacy the term rem means
    A. radiations per millisecond
    B. radiations.per minute
    C. roentgen-equivalent-man
    D. external roentgens per minute
    E. roentgen exposure per minute

20. Azathioprine is used primarily as a(an)
    A. tranquilizer
    B. cardiotonic
    C. immunosuppressive drug
    D. antidote
    E. antihypertensive

21. Phenol is
    A. soluble in water
    B. partially miscible in water
    C. a carboxylic acid
    D. red in color
    E. none of the above

22. ph is
    A. not temperature dependent
    B. a measure of acidity
    C. the same as pOH
    D. high for acids
    E. none of the above

23. Which of the following types of tissues frequently store drugs?
    A. Fatty tissue
    B. Muscle tissue
    C. Protein tissue
    D. A and B
    E. A and C

24. What is usually the first evidence that a drug is being stored in tissue?
    A. Small apparent volume of distribution
    B. Large apparent volume of distribution
    C. Decrease of drug in urine
    D. Decrease of metabolites in urine
    E. Marked side effects

25. Oxytocin is used to
    A. treat hypogonadism
    B. induce labor
    C. raise blood pressure
    D. prevent conception
    E. treat amenorrhea

26. Which of the following drugs undergoes marked hydrolysis in the GI tract?
    A. Aspirin
    B. Penicillin G
    C. Tylenol
    D. Hydrocortisone
    E. Chlortetracycline

27. Surface-active agents tend to enhance absorption due to
    A. effects on biological membrane
    B. effects on dissolution rate of drugs
    C. reduction of interfacial tension
    D. B and C
    E. A, B, and C

28. Which of the following imparts a pale blue fluorescence to urine following administration?
    A. Triamterene
    B. Cascara
    C. Riboflavin
    D. Azogantrisin
    E. Nitrofurantoin

29. What effect does plasma-protein binding have on biotransformation?
    A. None
    B. Changes the mechanism
    C. Prevents formation of metabolites
    D. Slows the process
    E. Speeds up the process

30. Celestone soluspan combines two salts of
    A. dexamethasone
    B. betamethasone
    C. cortisone
    D. prednisone
    E. prednisolone

31. The principal factor that makes enteric-coated tablets unpredictable in drug therapy is
    A. pH
    B. premature release of drug
    C. failure to release drug
    D. state of health of patient
    E. varying thickness of the coating

32. Carbolic acid is
    A. benzoic acid
    D. aspirin
    C. phenol
    D. salicylic acid
    E. none of the above

Match the drug with a prominent interaction:

A. Phenytoin
B. Alcoholic beverages
C. Digitoxin
D. Halothane
E. Urea

33. Sulfonylureas
34. Methadone
35. Cyclizine
36. Pancuronium bromide
37. Lithium salts

38. The advantage of foamtabs is primarily
A. better stability
B. faster absorption
C. improved solubility
D. improved taste
E. increased tablet hardness

39. Sterility tests for molds and yeasts should be conducted with
A. Thioglycollate medium
B. agar plates
C. honey medium
D. glucose broth
E. none of the above

40. Solutions that contain bacteriostatic agents
A. cannot be tested for sterility
B. must be cultured on agar plates for sterility tests
C. must be diluted beyond the bacteriostatic level for sterility tests
D. do not require a sterility test
E. none of the above

41. The sterility test for liquids involves
    A. colorimetric assay
    B. rabbit test
    C. injection into guinea pigs
    D. culturing in fluid thioglycollate medium
    E. none of the above

42. Oral hypoglycemic agents increase the metabolism of
    A. propanolol
    B. penicillins
    C. lidocaine
    D. digitoxin
    E. morphine

43. Strong iodine solution contains KI for the purpose of
    A. preservation
    B. reducing agent
    C. preventing precipitation
    D. increasing potency
    E. none of the above

44. Organic nitrates are not very useful in acute angina attacks because they
    A. are insoluble
    B. can only be given orally
    C. cause very servere side effects
    D. only mask the symptoms
    E. must be biconverted before being active

45. The adult dose of a drug is 6 gr. What dose should be given to a 6-year-old child according to Young's rule?
    A. 195 mg
    B. 10 mg
    C. 65 mg
    D. 10 mg
    E. 130 mg

46. Why does the USP state that morphine SO_4 must be kept in tight light-resistant containers?
    A. It loses water to the air
    B. It takes up water from the air
    C. It oxidizes slowly in air
    D. It takes up CO_2
    E. It volatilizes in air

47. A source of anticarcinogenic drugs is
   A. belladonna
   B. nux vomica
   C. vinca rosea
   D. cascara
   E. digitalis

48. An Rx calls for 30 cc of a 1:500 solution of zinc sulfate. Which of the following methods does NOT provide the proper amount of zinc sulfate required?
   A. 2 ophthalmic tablets of zinc sulfate containing 1 grain per tablet
   B. 4.0 cc of a stock solution 1:60 zinc sulfate
   C. 1 dram of a solution containg 8 gr/fl oz
   D. 2 tablets containing 0.030 g of zinc sulfate per tablet
   E. All provide the proper amount

49. If a CNS drug is extensively ionized at the pH of blood it will
   A. penetrate the blood-brain barrier slowly
   B. penetrate the blood-brain barrier rapidly
   C. not penetrate the blood-brain barrier
   D. be eleiminated slowly
   E. not be distributed to any tissue sites

50. In situ salt formation is a technique used in drug therapy to overcome
   A. lack of solubility of salt
   B. complexation problems
   C. poor absorption
   D. chemical instability
   E. none of the above

51. Pharmacists should caution patients who are taking niacin that this drug
   A. stains the urine bright red
   B. causes ringing in the ears
   C. causes muscular weakness
   D. should be taken before meals
   E. should be taken with meals

52. If a drug has a biological half-life of 6.9 days, the best dosing interval would be
    A. weekly
    B. biweekly
    C. semiweekly
    D. qid
    E. daily

53. Tween 20 is a
    A. deflocculant
    B. lipophilic surfactant
    C. preservative
    D. hydrophilic surfactant
    E. none of the above

54. Which of the following factors does NOT influence the rate of absorption from solutions to any significant extent?
    A. Biological half-life
    B. Viscosity
    C. Reversible complexation
    D. Micellular solubilization
    E. Chemical stability

55. First order half-life is equal to
    A. 1/k
    B. k
    C. 0.693/k
    D. 2 k + 1
    E. none of the above

56. The purpose of parabens in syrups is as
    A. solubilizers
    B. preservatives
    C. buffers
    D. tonicity adjusters
    E. thickeners

57. Which of the following is NOT regarded as a narcotic?
    A. Dionin
    B. Meperidine
    C. Morphine
    D. Codeine
    E. Propoxyphene

58. Brij is a trade name for a
    A. suspending agent
    B. surfactant
    C. deflocculant
    D. propellant
    E. flavor

59. Hemin (Panhematin) is derived from
    A. vitamin B_{12}
    B. red blood cells
    C. ferrous sulfate
    D. ferric compounds
    E. the liver

60. A substance used frequently to polish tablets is
    A. sodium chloride
    B. lactose
    C. air-dried talc
    D. starch
    E. calcium chloride

61. Sodium lauryl sulfate is a(an)
    A. alcohol
    B. ketone
    C. deflocculant
    D. wetting agent
    E. preservative

62. A prescription calls for 25 mM of potassium chloride. How many grams of KCl (MW 74.6) are needed?
    A. 7.46 g
    B. 0.746 g
    C. 8.86 g
    D. 1.86 g
    E. 0.186 g

63. An IV order requires 5 million units of sodium penicillin G to be added to 1 liter of normal saline. How many mEq of sodium are available per liter of solution?
    A. 154
    B. 1540
    C. 8.4
    D. 162
    E. 1620

64. Which is NOT correct?
   A. Chloramphenicol is well absorbed by the oral route and diffuses well into tissues
   B. Solutions more alkaline than pH 9-9.5 are not stable and are rapidly destroyed
   C. Rectal doses of chloramphenicol for infants should be greater than oral
   D. Chloramphenicol is devoid of toxicity and is well tolerated
   E. An afebrile period follows administration of chloramphenicol in certain conditions

65. An order calls for 500 ml of a solution of potassium sulfate to be made so that it contains 10 mEq of K_+. How many grams of potassium sulfate are required?
   A. 0.440
   B. .4.44
   C. 0.044
   D. 0.870
   E. 8.70

66. How many milliliters of a 10% KCl (MW 74.6) solution contain 5.0 mEq of K_+?
   A. 2.10
   B. 21.0
   C. 3.73
   D. 37.3
   E. 0.373

67. Gamma globulin fraction is separated from serum by
   A. centrifugation
   B. filtration
   C. dialysis
   D. salting out
   E. agglutination

68. An advantage of cyclacillin (Cyclapen-W) over ampicillin is
   A. it has a broader spectrum
   B. it produces a lower incidence of diarrhea
   C. it may be given orally
   D. it is more stable
   E. it is less expensive

69. Hashish is directly related to
    A. opium
    B. heroin
    C. marijuana
    D. LSD
    E. mescaline

70. Patients taking carisoprodol (Rela) should be cautioned
    A. not to drive
    B. not to drink alcoholic beverages
    C. to increase fluid intake markedly
    D. to decrease salt intake
    E. none of the above

71. Tetracyclines tend to form complexes with
    A. calcium ions
    B. magnesium ions
    C. cluminum ions
    D. iron ions
    E. all of the above

72. Most drugs are
    A. strong electrolytes
    B. weak electrolytes
    C. nonelectrolytes
    D. highly ionic
    E. none of the above

73. The major mechanism of degradation of drugs in the GI tract is
    A. oxidation
    B. hydrolysis
    C. acetylation
    D. conjugation
    E. reduction

74. Sodium polystyrene sulfonate (Kayexelate) is used for
    A. reducing elevated potassium levels
    B. softening the stool
    C. reducing gas
    D. treating scabies
    E. treating ulcers

75. An isotonic solution is one which
   A. does not cause hemolysis
   B. has same salt compositon of plasma
   C. does not cause crenulation
   D. causes crenulation
   E. has a freezing point less than that of plasma

76. Hyaluronidase has been used as an adjunct to
   A. prevent oxidation of drugs
   B. increase absorption of injected drugs
   C. prevent fluid loss
   D. speed detoxication by enzyme induction
   E. produce sustained action

77. The buffer equation is also known as
   A. Young's equation
   B. Charles' law
   C. Henderson-Hasselbalch equation
   D. Stokes' law
   E. none of the above

78. The pKw of water at 25° C is
   A. 7
   B. 14
   C. 1×10^{-14}
   D. 1×10^{-7}
   E. 1

79. Edetate disodium (Endrate) is used primarily to lower levels of
   A. sodium
   B. potassium
   C. calcium
   D. lithium
   E. uric acid

80. For which of the following drugs is biotransformation essential for therapeutic activity?
   A. Methanol
   B. Ethyl alcohol
   C. Phenacetin
   D. Aspirin
   E. Penicllin G

81. USP acetylsalicylic acid tablets should be packaged and stored in
   A. well-closed containers
   B. tightly closed containers
   C. light-resistant containers
   D. tightly closed, light-resistant containers
   E. none of the above

82. Benzalkonium chloride solution is partially inactivated by
   A. soap
   B. warming the solution
   C. methyl cellulose
   D. acetone
   E. none of the above

83. The usual purpose of chilling medication prior to administration is to increase
   A. absorption
   B. palatability
   C. stability
   D. ionization
   E. gastric motility

84. A route or method of administration for drugs which distribute poorly is
   A. IM
   B. IV infusion
   C. tissue implant
   D. SC
   E. intracerebral

85. A chromogen is
   A. associated with heredity
   B. a certified dye
   C. a precursor of color
   D. a dye fixative
   E. a colored substance

86. How many grams of aspirin must be dissolved in 484 cc of alcohol to make a 12% solution?
    A. 76
    B. 66
    C. 112
    D. 48
    E. 58

Match the following dose forms with a primary advantage of each:

A. Sustained action
B. Rapid solubility
C. Tamper proof
D. Metered dose
E. Improved

87. Sublingual tablets
88. Kapseals
89. Repetabs
90. Medihaler
91. Effervescent salts

92. Needle-shaped crystals are frequently formed on the surface of aspirin on long standing due to decomposition. The substance formed is
    A. C_6H_4 (OH) COOH
    B. CH_3 COOH
    C. C_6H_4 (OCH_3) COOH
    D. C_6H_5OH
    E. $C_6H_4(OH)_2$

93. Keesom forces occur between
    A. dipoles
    B. induced dipoles
    C. ions
    D. ions and dipoles
    E. ions and induced dipoles

94. Ranitidine is used primarily to treat
    A. staphylococcal infections
    B. diarrhea
    C. infant colic
    D. trigeminal neuralgia
    E. ulcers

95. A robengatope is a radioisotope used primarily to test
   A. brain function
   B. kidney function
   C. liver function
   D. rate of excretion
   E. rate of drug absorption

96. A solvent which can either accept or donate protons is said to be
   A. aprotic
   B. amphiprotic
   C. proteolytic
   D. acidic
   E. basic

97. Glycerin suppositories contain 92% glycerin and are solidified by the use of
   A. white wax
   B. stearic acid
   C. sodium stearate
   D. PEG 4000
   E. glyceryl triacetate

98. When silver nitrate decomposes by oxidation it gives
   A. a red precipitate
   B. a white precipitate
   C. a darkened solution
   D. a green color
   E. no visible change

99. The K term in the biological half-life equations is a combination of
   A. Ke and Km
   B. Ka and Km
   C. Ka and Ke
   D. Ka, Km and Ke
   E. Ka - (Ke + Km)

100. Which of the following is NOT a major pathway or type of biotransformation?
   A. Oxidation
   B. Deamination
   C. Reduction
   D. Hydrolysis
   E. Conjugation

101. In dispensing Azogantrisin the pharmacist should warn the patient that
A. he is likely to get a rash
B. the drug can only be taken at night
C. the drug can only be taken in the morning
D. it colors the urine red
E. the drug should be taken with food

102. What is the major reason that animal studies are NOT infallible in predicting drug efficacy or toxicity?
A. Differences in biotransformation
B. Differences in elimination mechanism
C. Differences in distribution mechanisms
D. Differences in absorption mechanisms
E. Differences in average weights

103. Talcum powders are most effectively sterilized by
A. autoclave
B. dry heat
C. gas sterilization
D. millipore
E. freeze drying

104. Glycerin is used in the eye primarily
A. to constrict the pupil
B. to dilate the pupil
C. to clear corneal haze
D. as a contact lens solution
E. to prevent itching

105. Plastics are normally sterilized with
A. direct flame
B. oven heat
C. ethylene oxide
D. steam under pressure
E. steam under vacuum

106. Shrinkage of gels by extrusion of liquid is called
A. syneresis
B. coacervation
C. ebullition
D. dilatancy
E. plasticity

107. Compazine syrup
   A. is deliquescent
   B. is effervescent
   C. should be dispensed in its original container
   D. is hygroscopic
   E. should never be given to children

108. How many milliliters of concentrated HCl (37% w/w) with a specific gravity of 1.35 should be used to make 4 fluid ounces of a 5% (w/v) solution?
   A. 0.12 ml
   B. 120 ml
   C. 1.2 ml
   D. 9 ml
   E. 12 ml

109. The dose of a drug is 0.5 mg per kilogram. What dose should be given a child of 6 who weighs 44 lb?
   A. 0.003 g
   B. 0.033 g
   C. 0.010 g
   D. 0.100 g
   E. 0.05 g

Match each drug with its primary action:

   A. Antifoaming agent
   B. Fecal softener
   C. Relief of coughs
   D. Antidiarrheal
   E. Laxative

110. Simethicone (Mylicon)
111. Dextromethorphan
112. Docusate calcium (Surfak)
113. Psyllium (Serutan)
114. Loperimide (Imodium)

115. Oleic acid is
   A. a saturated fatty acid
   B. an unsaturated ketone
   C. photosensitive
   D. official as a salt
   E. an unsaturated fatty acid

116. Rancidity of a fat is due to
   A. oxidation
   B. reduction
   C. neutralization
   D. hydrolysis
   E. saponification

117. The minimal effective flow rate of air in laminar flow hoods should be not less than how many cubic feet per minute?
   A. 10
   B. 50
   C. 100
   D. 500
   E. 1000

118. Which of the following compounds of undecylenic acid is most commonly used in therapy?
   A. Zinc
   B. Magnesium
   C. Manganese
   D. Silver
   E. Mercury

119. A vitamin which stains the urine is
   A. vitamin D
   B. thiamine
   C. inositol
   D. riboflavin
   E. niacin

120. What effect does increased tissue storage have on biological half-life of drugs?
   A. Makes it erratic
   B. Renders it meaningless
   C. Decreases it
   D. Increases it
   E. None

121. A 30 volume peroxide corresponds to
   A. 3% by weight
   B. 30% by weight
   C. 30% by volume
   D. 9% by weight
   E. 99% by weight

122. The Munsell system is associated with
    A. flavor
    B. odor
    C. chemical classification
    D. color
    E. incompatibilities

123. The dose of a drug is 5 mg/kg of body weight. What dose should be given to a 110-lb woman?
    A. 2 gr
    B. 4 gr
    C. 500 mg
    D. 5 gr
    E. 0.5 gr

124. The two most common proteins involved in plasma-protein binding are
    A. barbiturates
    B. globulin and plasmin
    C. albumin and globulin
    D. fibrin and plasmin
    E. plasminogen and fibrin

125. Which of the following is classified as a loop diuretic?
    A. Urea
    B. Acetazolamide
    C. Triamterene
    D. Spironolactone
    E. Furosemide

126. Diuretics tend to enhance lithium salt toxicity due to
    A. sodium depletion
    B. potassium depletion
    C. direct drug interaction
    D. increased absorption
    E. increased solubility of the lithium salts

127. An oral antifungal agent is
    A. zinc undecylenate
    B. Tetrex
    C. Desenex
    D. griseofulvin
    E. Sopronol

128. A disadvantage of sodium saccharin as a sweetening agent is
   A. its bitter aftertaste
   B. its solubility in water
   C. its poor strength compared to glucose
   D. its poor strength compared to dulcin
   E. its toxicity

129. Responsibility for control of drugs covered by the drug abuse amendments falls upon
   A. DEA
   B. FTC
   C. FDA
   D. ICC
   E. none of the above

130. Nitrofurantoin (Furadantin) is most active when the pH of the urinary tract is
   A. neutral
   B. over 9.5
   C. between 6.0 and 7.0
   D. 5.5 or less
   E. none of the above

131. Iodine is soluble in water in the presence of
   A. sodium citrate
   B. sodium sulfate
   C. lactose
   D. PVP
   E. PEG

132. Povan could be classified as a
   A. deflocculant
   B. lubricant
   C. cyanine dye
   D. disintegrator
   E. surfactant

133. Aloes are used to treat
   A. burns
   B. gastritis
   C. blood dyscrasias
   D. carcinomas
   E. vertigo

134. The class of substances responsible for most accidental poisonings in children is
A. detergents
B. salicylate analgesics
C. bleaches
D. belladonna alkaloids
E. commercial dyes

135. Which of the following can cause discoloration of teeth?
A. Chloromycetin
B. Penicillin
C. Achromycin
D. Kanamycin
E. Sulfadiazine

136. Which of the following can increase the serum levels of penicillins significantly?
A. Salicylates
B. Probenicid
C. Antacids
D. Kaolin
E. Starches

137. Storage of soaking solutions for hard contact lenses should be
A. heated prior to use
B. acidified with weak acids
C. replaced weekly
D. replaced daily
E. none of the above

138. The prinicipal limiting factor in the rate of absorption from suspensions is
A. dissolution rate
B. viscosity
C. the suspending agent
D. chemical stability
E. physical stability

139. Which of the following diuretics is quite effective even in the presence of electrolyte or acid-base imbalance?
   A. Ethacrynic acid
   B. Ammonium chloride
   C. Chlorothiazide
   D. Acetazolamide
   E. None of the above

140. Ultrasonic waves have a frequency of
   A. 10-20 kc
   B. 20 kc or above
   C. 50 kc or above
   D. over 100 kc
   E. 80-90 kc

141. Which of the following solutions should be sterile when dispensed?
   A. Tinctures
   B. Ophthalmic solutions
   C. Spirits
   D. Syrups
   E. None of the above

142. Film coatings are
   A. enteric coatings
   B. sustained release
   C. very brittle
   D. very flexible
   E. very thick

143. A type of bond frequently seen in complexes is
   A. hydrogen bond
   B. ionic bond
   C. semipolar bond
   D. double bond
   E. triple bond

144. Which of the following agents may stain clothing when used topically?
   A. Zinc oxide
   B. Titanium dioxide
   C. PABA
   D. PAS
   E. Undecylenic acid

145. Radioactive decay follows a
    A. mixed order rate
    B. fractional order rate
    C. zero order rate
    D. first order rate
    E. second order rate

146. The HLB system is used to classify
    A. flavors
    B. colors
    C. surfactants
    D. organic ring structures
    E. perfumes

147. In situ salt formation usually occurs
    A. during in vivo distribution
    B. before absorption
    C. in storage sites
    D. after biotransformation
    E. in the kidney

148. Passive diffusion
    A. can operate against a concentration gradient
    B. is usually slow
    C. required high energy
    D. is usually quite fast
    E. requires low energy

149. Glucagon may be used as a diagnostic agent in radiographic examination of the
    A. bones
    B. GI tract
    C. liver
    D. kidney
    E. brain

150. A prevalent drug interaction of fluoride solutions involves
    A. eggs
    B. dairy products
    C. meats
    D. fish
    E. many vegetables

151. Ostwald pipettes are used to measure
   A. specific gravity
   B. samples for assay
   C. density
   D. osmotic pressure
   E. viscosity

152. Alpha particles are very similar to
   A. hydrogen atoms
   B. helium atoms
   C. neutrons
   D. protons
   E. electrons

153. Gamma rays are very similar to
   A. x-rays
   B. alpha radiation
   C. beta radiation
   D. neutrinos
   E. antineutrinos

154. A drug that reverses plasma-protein binding is often referred to as
   A. a protein hydrolysate
   B. a displacer
   C. a solvate
   D. a carrier substance
   E. an enzyme

155. Patients using selenium sulfide should be warned that it should NOT be
   A. used more than once a month
   B. applied to wet hair
   C. used after bleaching or tinting the hair
   D. rinsed from hair for 30 minutes
   E. used after soap shampoos

156. A rich source of vitamin A is
   A. lean meats
   B. bread
   C. liver
   D. poultry
   E. fish liver oils

157. Contact angle is used to measure
   A. moisture content of granules
   B. spreadability of ointments
   C. disintegration of tablets
   D. coefficient of friction of powders
   E. none of the above

158. According to Stokes law, the creaming of emulsions is indirectly proportional to
   A. density of the dispersed phase
   B. gravity
   C. radius of dispersed phase
   D. viscosity of the medium
   E. none of the above

159. Plasma levels of vitamin A may be significantly affected by
   A. vitamin D
   B. oral contraceptives
   C. cephalosporins
   D. aspirin
   E. Darvon-N

160. The most common disintegrator in compressed tablets is
   A. dextrose
   B. lactose
   C. starch
   D. potassium bitartrate
   E. powdered sucrose

161. Freons are
   A. alkanes
   B. alkenes
   C. alkynes
   D. fluorinated hydrocarbons
   E. mixture of CO_2 and air

162. Agglomeration of particles in emulsions is often called
   A. grouping
   B. coalescence
   C. dimerization
   D. polymerization
   E. dichromatism

163. Absorption of vitamin A from the GI tract depends on
   A. the presence of bile in the intestine
   B. which salt is used
   C. acid-base balance
   D. needs of the patient
   E. pH of the intestine

164. Purity rubric means
   A. purified coloring substance
   B. Pure Food and Drug Act
   C. USP or NF statement of required purity
   D. substance requires purification
   E. none of the above

165. Which of the following does NOT enhance complexation?
   A. Gums
   B. Cellulose derivatives
   C. Polyols
   D. Nonionic surfactants
   E. Quaternary ammonium compounds

166. Which of the following factors may make it necessary to give lower doses of drugs to geriatric patients?
   A. Reduction of enzyme activity
   B. Reduced kidney function
   C. Enhanced absorption
   D. A and B
   E. A, B, and C

167. A drug that is frequently administered by inhalation is
   A. insulin
   B. isoproterenol
   C. allopurinol
   D. penicillin
   E. nitroglycerin

168. FDA regulations requiring sealing of containers for OTC drugs resulted from contamination of Tylenol with
   A. arsenic
   B. cyanide
   C. sympathomimetics
   D. acids
   E. bacterial toxins

169. Methotrexate should never be used concurrently with
   A. penicillin
   B. meprobamate
   C. epinephrine
   D. ethinamate
   E. aspirin

170. Tablet hardness range is normally
   A. 0.2 - 0.5 kg
   B. 0.5 - 1.0 kg
   C. 1.0 - 2.0 kg
   D. 2.0 - 3.5 kg
   E. 3.5 - 7.0 kg

171. An antidote for heparin overdosage is
   A. protamine sulfate
   B. BAL
   C. atropine
   D. calcium salts
   E. dicumarol

172. Anticoagulent acid citrate dextrose injection is required to be pyrogen-free. Pyrogens are
   A. organic catalysts formed in living cells
   B. antigens contained in bacteria
   C. nonspecific globulins
   D. products which stimulate hematopoietic organs
   E. products causing febrile reaction upon injection

173 Weakly basic drugs are eliminated best under what conditions?
   A. Alkaline urine
   B. Acid urine
   C. Neutral urine
   D. Slowed biotransformation
   E. Lack of biotransformation

174 Oral hypoglycemics are usually most useful in
   A. juvenile diabetes
   B. labile diabetes
   C. brittle diabetes
   D. late-onset diabetes
   E. uncomplicated diabetes

175. Sulfinpyrazone (Antarane) frequently produces which of the following side effects?
   A. Headache
   B. Upper GI disturbances
   C. Ringing in the ears
   D. Respiratory depression
   E. Diarrhea

176. Amyl nitrite is usually administered
   A. by inhalation
   B. sublingually
   C. IM
   D. IV
   E. rectally

What is the average oral dose of each of the following?

   A. 5 mg/kg
   B. 100 mg
   C. 25 mg
   D. 0.75 mg
   E. 250 mg

177. Povan
178. Indocin
179. Dexamethasone
180. Erythromycin
181. Dilantin

182. Capsicum is used in OTC liniments
   A. to promote easy spreading
   B. for its odor
   C. to produce warmth or heat
   D. as an analgesic
   E. none of the above

183. Aluminum chloride is used mainly as a(an)
   A. antiemetic
   B. laxative
   C. suspending agent
   D. urinary acidifier
   E. antiperspirant

184. A substance that is often used to subcoat tablets is
   A. sugar
   B. carnauba wax
   C. shellac
   D. sodium stearate
   E. sodium chloride

185. Propranolol (Inderal) should be used only with extreme caution in patients suffering from
   A. depression
   B. cardiac arrhythmias
   C. hypertension
   D. hay fever
   E. diabetes

186. When prescribing oral contraceptives, a physician need NOT give special attention to women who have
   A. migraine headaches
   B. diabetes
   C. uterine tumors
   D. never had a pregnancy
   E. high blood pressure

Match the following generic names with the proper trade name:

A. Suavitil
B. Indocin
C. Placidyl
D. Neohydrin
E. Brevital
F. Valmid
G. Butazolidin
H. Thorazine
I. Ponstel
J. Vontrol

187. Mefenamic acid
188. Chloromerodrin
189. Benactyzine
190. Phenylbutazone
191. Chlorpromazine
192. Methohexital
193. Indomethacin
194. Ethchlorvynol
195. Ethinamate
196. Diphenidol

197. Why are nitroglycerin tablets relatively unstable?
   A. They become insoluble
   B. They are hygroscopic
   C. They are deliquescent
   D. The drug migrates from the tablets
   E. They tend to crumble

198. Antabuse is used to treat
   A. diabetes
   B. cholera
   C. alcoholism
   D. trench mouth
   E. mumps

199. Proposed changes in drug regulations must be published in which of the following to constitute official notice?
   A. Food and Drug Papers
   B. Congressional Record
   C. American Pharmaceutical Association Journal
   D. Federal Register
   E. All of the above

Match each drug with its prevalent use:

   A. Antidepressant
   B. Anticoagulant
   C. Antibiotic
   D. Analgesic
   E. Antineoplastic

200. Pantopon
201. Warfarin
202. Nortriptylene
203. Moxam
204. Cytarabine

205. Which of the following is available in a metered dose aerosol?
   A. Reserpine
   B. Isoproterenol
   C. Guanethidine
   D. Dimenhydramine
   E. Diphenylhydantoin

206. Benzoyl peroxide is used topically to treat
   A. skin carcinomas
   B. burns
   C. minor abrasions
   D. acne
   E. dermatitis

107. Adjustment of dosage of diphenylhydantoin is based primarily on
   A. patient response
   B. blood levels
   C. rate of excretion
   D. body weight
   E. prothrombin time

108. Darvon-N contains which of the following amounts of dextropropoxyphene napsylate?
   A. 50 mg
   B. 100 mg
   C. 32 mg
   D. 65 mg
   E. None of the above

209. Which of the following best describes Schedule I drugs?
   A. Most were formerly schedule A drugs
   B. No accepted medical use in the U.S.
   C. Used to be called exempt narcotics
   D. Potent analgesics used to treat pain
   E. Little potential for abuse

210. Which of the following is contraindicated with MAO inhibitors?
   A. Milk
   B. Cheeses
   C. Cola beverages
   D. Meats
   E. Fish

Match the following:

A. Chloral hydrate
B. Demethylchlortetracycline
C. Cyclizine
D. Amphetamine
E. Norethindrone

211. Marezine
212. Declomycin
213. Noctec
214. Biphetamine
215. Ortho-novum

216. Which of the following is NOT an advantage of aerosol dose forms?
A. Fine particle size
B. Easy to apply
C. Inexpensive
D. Even application
E. Less contamination

217. Which of the following may be used as plasma expanders?
A. Sodium salts
B. Dextrans
C. Starches
D. Calcium salts
E. Prostaglandins

218. Aerosols should be stored at temperatures of
A. 37°C or less
B. below 120°F
C. below 95°F
D. below 100°F
E. 25°C or less

219. A prescription calls for 500 mg of digoxin dissolved in enough solvent to make 3 fluid ounces. How much of this solution will contain approximately 1/30 gr of digoxin?
A. 5 minims
B. 4 minims
C. 8 minims
D. 10 minims
E. 6 minims

220. Which of the following should be stored in dark glass bottles?
A. Silver nitrate solution
B. Lime water
C. Syrup U.S.P.
D. Simple elixir
E. Coca-cola syrup

221. An antiemetic that contains principally carbohydrate derivatives is
A. Vesprin
B. Compazine
C. Tigan
D. Thorazine
E. Emetrol

222. Which of the following is used to offset the effects of coumarin derivatives?
A. Protamine sulfate
B. Adrenalin
C. Vitamin K
D. Calcium
E. BAL

223. Penicillamine is often calssified as a(an)
A. antioxidant
B. chelating agent
C. micelle
D. surfactant
E. humectant

224. Prostaglandin E_2 is used in the form of
   A. tablets
   B. capsules
   C. solutions
   D. vaginal suppositories
   E. IV injections

225. Most volatile oils are rich in
   A. terpenes
   B. sulfur-containing compounds
   C. fluorinated hydrocarbons
   D. glucocorticoids
   E. pyrimidines

226. A common evidence of deterioration of citrate of magnesia is
   A. darkening of color
   B. development of sour odor
   C. precipitation
   D. build up of excessive gas
   E. lightening of color

227. Opium is obtained by
   A. slitting capsules of a plant
   B. extraction from leaves of a plant
   C. grinding a plant
   D. chemical synthesis
   E. molecular modification

228. Tetrahydrazoline is used as a(an)
   A. eyeglass protectant
   B. contact lens solution
   C. mitotic
   D. mydriatic
   E. ocular decongestant

229. Which of the following statistical techniques is(are) useful for clinical trials?
   A. F test
   B. Chi Square test
   C. Latin Square
   D. A and B
   E. All of the above

230. Which of the following is NOT used as a binder for tablets?
   A. Talc
   B. Starch
   C. Glucose
   D. Sucrose
   E. Gelatin

Match the following:

   A. Nembutal
   B. Kaopectate
   C. Selsun
   D. Neosynephrine
   E. Tridione

231. Kaolin and pectin
232. Trimethadione
233. Pentobarbital
234. Selenium sulfide
235. Phenylephrine

236. GMP regulations (USFDA) apply primarily to
   A. controlled drugs
   B. wholesalers
   C. pharmaceutical manufacturers
   D. hospital pharmacy
   E. community pharmacy

237. pH is equivalent to pka at
   A. pH of 7
   B. pH of 1
   C. pH of 14
   D. half neutralization point
   E. neutralization point

238. A method for removing pyrogens from water involves
   A. oxidation with permanganate
   B. oxidation with H_2O_2
   C. precipitation with H_2S
   D. absorption on certain asbestos filter pads
   E. none of the above

239. Splitting off of the face of a tablet is called
  A. capping
  B. fissuring
  C. slugging
  D. whiskering
  E. picking

240. An instrument used to measure durability of tablets to shock and abrasion is a
  A. tensiometer
  B. dart penetrometer
  C. chilsomator
  D. brittleometer
  E. friabilator

241. Titanium dioxide is used primarily as a
  A. preservative
  B. tablet hardener
  C. sunscreen
  D. surfactant
  E. deflocculant

242. The nonaqueous vehicle used in injections is
  A. alcohol
  B. glycerol
  C. alcholic sodium stearate
  D. vegetable oils
  E. wax or liquid petrolatum

243. Which of the following drugs is commonly used to treat schistosomiasis?
  A. Methylene blue
  B. Praziquantel (Biltricide)
  C. Emetine HCl
  D. Chloroquine (Aralen)
  E. Oxytetracycline (Terramycin)

244. Most tests of statistical significance are based on the
  A. null hypothesis
  B. mean
  C. standard deviation
  D. range
  E. Chi Square test

245. An advantage of allopurinol (Zyloprin) over many uricosuric drugs is that it
   A. is far less toxic
   B. is more stable
   C. is faster acting
   D. may be given with salicylate analgesics
   E. is considerably less expensive

246. Chlorambucil (Leukeran) acts primarily as a(an)
   A. antibiotic
   B. mitotic inhibitor
   C. alkylating agent
   D. antimetabolite
   E. synthetic hormone

247. The equation for a straight line is $a = mx + b$. M represents the
   A. initial value of x
   B. slope of the line
   C. intercept with the y axis
   D. intercept with the x axis
   E. initial value of y

248. The boiling point of alcohol is 78°C. The corresponding temperature in degrees Fahrenheit is
   A. 46
   B. 10
   C. 172
   D. 156
   E. 140

249. For ophthalmic use, boric acid solution should be
   A. diluted with an equal volume of distilled water
   B. undiluted
   C. diluted with an equal volume of isotonic saline solution
   D. diluted with an equal volume of sterile distilled water
   E. diluted with an equal volume of sterile isotonic saline solution

250. Which of the following may stain the body and clothing?
   A. Meprobamate
   B. Benadryl
   C. Povan
   D. Kaopectate
   E. Acidulin

251. Valproic acid capsules if chewed will cause
   A. irritation of the mouth and throat
   B. destruction of the drug
   C. staining of the teeth
   D. hyperventilation
   E. blurring of the vision

252. Which of the following is NOT a side effect of cimetidine (Tagamet)?
   A. Neutropenia
   B. Dizziness
   C. Rash
   D. Constipation
   E. All of the above are side effects

253. In Stokes' law
   A. rate of settling is directly proportional to particle diameter
   B. viscosity is directly proportional to particle diameter
   C. temperature is important
   D. concentration of suspended phase in unimportant
   E. none of the above

254. A popular theory of acids and bases is
   A. Boyle's law
   B. Four Humors' theory
   C. Pythagorean theory
   D. Bronsted-Lowry theory
   E. Henry's theory

255. Salicyclic acid is used primarily as a(an)
   A. analgesic
   B. antipyretic
   C. cough suppressant
   D. uricosuric agent
   E. keratolytic agent

256. Spectinomycin (Trobicin) is used primarily to treat
   A. skin infections
   B. eye infections
   C. upper respiratory infections
   D. urinary tract infections
   E. gonorrhea

257. Preserved water is made by adding which of the following to purified water?
   A. Phenol
   B. Benzoic acid
   C. Zephiran
   D. Parabens
   E. None of the above

258. Which of the following acids is normally found in the liquid state in nature?
   A. Lactic acid
   B. Tartaric acid
   C. Benzoic acid
   D. Barbituric acid
   E. Salicylic acid

259. Which of the following is an expectorant agent?
   A. Codeine
   B. Dextromethorphan
   C. Glyceryl guaiacolate
   D. Glycerin
   E. Wild cherry syrup

260. A primary disadvantage of cool air vaporizes is
   A. discomfort
   B. noise
   C. staining properties
   D. lack of effectiveness
   E. no automatic shut-off

261. Veegum is a(an)
   A. polyol
   B. organic gum
   C. synthetic gum
   D. clay
   E. nonionic surfactant

262. The most prevalent adverse reaction of selenium sulfide is
   A. dryness of scalp
   B. oiliness of hair
   C. discoloration of hair
   D. loss of hair
   E. irritation of skin

263. A disadvantage of chloral hydrate is
   A. lack of absorption
   B. rapid elimination
   C. lack of chemical stability
   D. allergic reactions
   E. disagreeable odor

264. A common contaminant of either USP is
   A. ethanol
   B. methanol
   C. ketones
   D. peroxides
   E. heavy metals

265. The Crocker-Henderson system is used to classify
   A. flavors
   B. dyes
   C. odors
   D. surfactants
   E. deflocculants

266. Simethicone relieves flatulence primarily because of which of the following properties?
   A. Analgesic
   B. Laxative
   C. Fecal softening
   D. Defoaming action
   E. Foaming action

267. Econazole nitrate (Spectazole) is most effective against
   A. gram-negative bacteria
   B. viruses
   C. rickettsia
   D. fungal infestations
   E. tape worm

268. An aqueous solution of aluminum chloride is
    A. neutral
    B. acid
    C. alkaline
    D. amphoteric
    E. none of the above

Match each drug with the appropriate use:

    A. Topical antifungal
    B. Diuretic
    C. Antidepressant
    D. Arthritis treatment
    E. Antiasthmatic

269. Desipramine (Norpramin)
270. Acrisorcin (Acrinol)
271. Tolmetin (Tolectin)
272. Cromolyn Sodium
273. Polythiazide (Renese)

274. Pyrivinium pamoate (Povan) dosage is usually adjusted according to
    A. age
    B. biological half-life
    C. prothrombin time
    D. physiological state
    E. body weight

275. Which of the following is contained in a number of sun-tanning lotions?
    A. Benzocaine
    B. PABA
    C. Zinc oxide
    D. Benzoic acid
    E. Salicylic acid

276. Lente insulin is
    A. given only intravenously
    B. 70% crystalline, 30% amorphous insulin
    C. 30% crystalline, 70% amorphous insulin
    D. another name for NPH insulin
    E. the shortest-acting insulin preparation

Match the following:

A. Soluble in water, suitable for IV use
B. Acidic solutions rapidly deteriorate
C. Useful for extemporaneous preparations

277. Erythromycin
278. Erythromycin ethyl carbonate
279. Erythromycin glucoheptonate

280. Diuril is
A. a carbonic anhydrase inhibitor
B. a mercurial diuretic
C. a nonmercurial diuretic
D. a uricosuric agent
E. none of the above

281. Probenecid should NOT be used in the treatment of gout in conjunction with salicylates because
A. the toxicity of probenecid is increased by the acidic salicylates
B. probenecid is not effective in gout
C. therapeutic actions are antagonistic
D. their actions are synergistic
E. none of the above

Match the following:

A. Vioform
B. Doriden
C. Terramycin
D. Valmid
E. Placidyl
F. Temaril
G. Librium

282. Trimeprazine
283. Glutethimide
284. Ethinamate
285. Iodochlorhydroxyquin
286. Chlordiazepoxide
287. Ethchlorvynol
288. Oxytetracycline

289. The usual concentration of KCl in hyperalimentation fluids is
   A. 1 g/l
   B. 2 g/l
   C. 1 mEq/l
   D. 4 mEq/l
   E. 40 mEq/l

Match the following:

   A. Medihaler
   B. Glosset
   C. Abboject
   D. Gradumet
   E. Medilet

290. Long-release tablet
291. Sublingual tablet
292. Aerosol device
293. Color-flecked tablet
294. Disposable syringe

295. Ipsatol contains which of the following as an expectorant?
   A. Ammonium chloride
   B. Ipecac
   C. Glyceryl guaiacolate
   D. Potassium iodide
   E. None of the above

296. All tetracycline antibiotics
   A. have the same chemical structures but are stereoisomers
   B. are destroyed by alkali hydroxides
   C. produce the same incidence of side effects
   D. are isolated from streptococcus rinosus
   E. all of the above

297. Which of the following is used topically as a cardiovascular agent?
   A. Propranolol
   B. Procainamide
   C. Digoxin
   D. Nitroglycerin
   E. Lidocaine

298. Aminocaproic acid is used to treat
   A. warts
   B. hemorrhage
   C. hypertension
   D. protein loss
   E. ulcers

299. The concentration of nitrofurazone solutions used ophthalmically is
   A. 2%
   B. 20%
   C. 0.02%
   D. 5%
   E. 1%

300. DMSO is no longer used clinically because it was found to produce
   A. agranulocytosis
   B. skin damage
   C. brain damage
   D. eye damage
   E. carcinomas

301. The ideal antiseptic concentration of ethyl alcohol is
   A. 95%
   B. 70%
   C. 100%
   D. 50%
   E. 75%

302. Which of the following is NOT metabolized by the liver?
   A. Phenobarbital
   B. Barbital
   C. Pentobarbital
   D. Allobarbital
   E. Secobarbital

303. Vancomycin is
   A. isolated from a strain of bacillus
   B. well absorbed orally
   C. preferably administered IV
   D. preferably administered IM
   E. a single chemical entity

304. Pyridoxine is
   A. vitamin B_6
   B. vitamin A
   C. vitamin B_1
   D. vitamin K
   E. vitamin D

Match the following:

   A. Chloromycetin
   B. Novobiocin
   C. Streptomycin
   D. Vancomycin
   E. Erythromycin

305. S. venezuelae
306. S. erythreus
307. S. orientalis
308. S. niveus
309. S. griseus

310. Which of the following is the most effective sun-screen?
   A. PABA
   B. Titanium dioxide
   C. Methoxysoralen
   D. Menthyl salicylate
   E. Baby oil

Match the following:

A. Multiple vitamin
B. Cough syrup
C. Poison ivy therapy
D. Diarrhea control
E. Motion sickness
F. Hemorrhoids
G. Antacid
H. Antiseptic
I. Cold therapy
J. Laxative

311. Contac
312. Maalox
313. Formula 44
314. Dramamine
315. Caligesic
316. Unicap
317. Kaopectate
318. Glycerin suppositories
319. Anusol
320. Merthiolate

321. Tuinal (Lilly) contains amobarbital and
A. pentobarbital
B. phenobarbital
C. secobarbital
D. aspirin
E. caffeine

322. Which of the following drugs is used to treat fungal infestations of the eye?
A. Nafcillin
B. Idoxurine (Idu)
C. Natamycin (Natacyn)
D. Cephizoxime (Cefizox)
E. Amikacin (Amikin)

323. What imparts the pink color to calamine?
   A. Zinc oxide
   B. Titanium dioxide
   C. Ferric oxide
   D. Carmine
   E. FDC red no. 3

Match each substance with its chief pharmaceutical use:

A. Flavoring agent
B. Ointment base
C. Coloring agent
D. Antioxidant
E. Aerosol propellant
F. Suspending agent
G. Binder for tablets
H. Diluent
I. Solvent
J. Lubricant
K. Suppository base
L. Buffering agent

324 Freon
325 Sodium metabisulfite
326. Amaranth
327. Erhyl acetate
328. Acacia
329. Petrolatum
330. Alcohol U.S.P.
331. Lactose
332. Theobroma oil
333. Starch paste
334. Magnesium stearate
335. Potassium metaphosphate

336. Glycerin has a specific gravity of 1.25. One gallon weighs
   A. 591.25 g
   B. 473 g
   C. 4730 g
   D. 128 g
   E. 4800 g

Match the following:

A. 64.8 mg
B. 128 fl oz
C. 60 min
D. 60 gr
E. 473 ml
F. 16.23 min
G. 454 g
H. None of the above

337. 1 fluid dram
338. 1 pint
339. 1 milliliter
340. 1 grain
341. 1 gallon
342. 1 apothecary dram
343. 1 pound

Match each substance with its primary action in cold or cough preparations:

A. Analgesic-antipyretic
B. Expectorant
C. Moisturizer
D. Decongestant
E. Antitussive

344. Phenylpropanolamine
345. Dextromethorphan
346. Glycerin
347. Acetaminophen
348. Guaifenesin

349. Tinctures
A. are made by direct solution of a volatile oil
B. represent 100 g of drug of 100 ml of finished tincture
C. are aqueous solutions of active constituents of drugs
D. are sweetened, flavored aqueous alcoholic solutions of drugs
E. none of the above

350. Vitamin K is associated with
   A. pellagra
   B. nerves
   C. hemoglobin concentration
   D. bones
   E. blood clotting

351. Which of the following is found in vitamin B_{12}?
   A. Magnesium
   B. Nickel
   C. Iron
   D. Cobalt
   E. Manganese

Match each drug with its usual route of administration:

   A. Drops in eye
   B. Topical
   C. By inhalation
   D. Intramuscular
   E. Intravaginal

352. Isoptofrin
353. Mycostatin
354. Isoetharine
355. Selenium sulfide
356. Immune globulin

Match each active ingredient with the appropriate product containing this ingredient:

   A. Collodion
   B. Rubbing alcohol
   C. Ascorbic acid injection
   D. Hydrophilic petrolatum
   E. Enteric-coated tablets

357. Sodium metabisulfite
358. Cholesterol
359. Methylisobutylketone
360. Cellulose acetate phthalate
361. Pyroxylin

Match each drug with the appropriate dosage, dosage range, or strength:

A. 50-150 mg
B. 65 mg
C. 15-30 mg
D. 25,000-50,000 international units
E. 5 mg per kg of body weight
F. 125-750 mg per day
G. 2% topical
H. 0.5 to 1.5 mg
I. 0.5 to 1.0 mg per kg
J. 0.3 to 0.4 mcg

362. Meperidine
363. Dextropropoxyphene
364. Codeine
365. Vitamin D
366. Pyrivinium pamoate
367. Levodopa
368. Stannous fluoride
369. Digoxin
370. Doxapram
371. Vitamin B_{12}

Match the following:

A. Antihistaminic
B. Migraine therapy
C. Cough preparation
D. Vaginal antifungal
E. Muscle relaxant
F. Non-narcotic analgesic
G. Antipruritic
H. Antiarthritic
I. Antiemetic
J. Mood elevator
K. Diagnostic for myasthenia gravis
L. Diuretic
M. Anticonvulsant

372. Talwin
373. Temaril
374. Indocin
375. Tensilon
376. Quelidrine
377. Benadryl
378. Compazine syrup
379. Robaxin
380. Sansert
381. Tridione
382. Naqua
383. Elavil
384. AVC cream

Match each of the OTC drugs with its proper class:

A. External analgesic
B. Eye wash
C. Antidiarrheal
D. Sleep aid
E. Internal analgesic
F. Toothache remedy
G. Cough preparation
H. Diet food
I. Burn remedy
J. Laxative
K. Treat hemorrhoids
L. Antacid
M. Poison ivy remedy

385. Kao-Con
386. Sominex
387. Actifed
388. Metrecal
389. Orajel
390. Riopan
391. Musterole
392. Solarcaine
393. Preparation H
394. Collyrium
395. Ziradryl
396. Kondremul
397. Tempra

398. Another name for polyethylene glycol polymers is
   A. sodium alginate
   B. silica gel
   C. carbowax
   D. Friar paste
   E. none of the above

399. PEG 4000 monostearate is NOT miscible with
   A. water
   B. alcohol
   C. ether
   D. benzene
   E. isopropyl alcohol

Match the following:

   A. Every hour
   B. According to the art
   C. Before meals
   D. Mix
   E. Carbonated water
   F. With
   G. A powder
   H. A large spoonful
   I. A drop
   J. Make
   K. Dust
   L. If necessary
   M. As directed
   N. Immediately

400. $\bar{c}$
401. coch. mag.
402. pulv.
403. omn. hor.
404. s. a.
405. ft.
406. M.
407. a. c.
408. s. o. s.
409. Ag. aeratq.
410. ut dict.
411. gtt.
412. stat.
413. consperg.

Match the following:

A. Right eye
B. Left eye
C. A teaspoonful
D. Every other day
E. Four times a day before meals and at bedtime
F. Both eyes
G. Give four such doses
H. Without
I. As directed
J. When necessary

414. O. S.
415. q. i. d. a. c. et h. s.
416. pro re nata
417. O. D.
418. coch. parv.
419. O. U.
420. d. t. d. no. IV
421. Dieb. alt.
422. e. m. p.
423. s̄

424. The hydrogen ion concentration of a solution with a pH of 5.6 is
A. 3.9×10^{-5}
B. 2.5×10^{-6}
C. 2.5×10^{-5}
D. 7.0×10
E. 7.0×10^{-5}

425. An ophthalmic preparation should have which of the following pHs to conform to that of lacrimal fluid?
A. 6.2-6.8
B. 7.2-8.0
C. 8.4-9.0
D. 9.2-10
E. None of the above

Match the following:

A. Paradione
B. Coumadin
C. Compazine
D. Desenex
E. Fungizone
F. Dopar
G. Neutrapen
H. Serpasil
I. Hedulin
J. Polycillin
K. Gantrisin
L. Santyl

426. Zinc undecylenate
427. Paramethadione
428. L-Dopa
429. Warfarin
430. Phenindione
431. Prochlorperazine
432. Amphotericin B
433. Sulfisoxazole
434. Penicillinase
435. Reserpine
436. Ampicillin
437. Collagenase

438. How many milliliters of a 5% stock solution should be used to prepare 4 fluid ounces of a 1:200 solution?
A. 48 ml
B. 10 ml
C. 4 ml
D. 1.2 ml
E. 12 ml

439. A solution is prepared by dissolving a 1-ounce package of drug in 1 fluid ounce of water. What is the % w/v of the resulting solution?
A. 100%
B. 50%
C. 48.6%
D. 46.5%
E. 33.3%

440. Indomethacin should be used with extra care in patients suffering from
A. infections
B. bursitis
C. gout
D. acne
E. burns

441. -12°C is equivalent to
A. 36°F
B. 12°F
C. 10.4°F
D. 5°F
E. -2°F

442. One tablespoon is approximately equivalent to
A. 15 ml
B. 10 ml
C. 8 ml
D. 20 ml
E. 30 ml

Match the following:

A. Vibramycin
B. Cotazym
C. Banthine
D. Hygroton
E. Betalin
F. Doriden
G. Skelaxin
H. Pronestyl
I. Tegretol
J. Kenalog
K. Ilotycin
L. Thorazine
M. Rondomycin
N. Furacin
O. Valium

443. Doxycycline
444. Pancreolipase
445. Methacycline
446. Carbamazepine
447. Diazepam
448. Metaxolone
449. Methantheline
450. Nitrofurazone
451. Triamcinolone
452. Procainamide
453. Glutethimide
454. Thiamine
455. Erythromycin
456. Chlorthalidone
457. Vitamin B_1

458. In streptococcal infections, penicillins should be continued for
   A. 15 days
   B. 10 days
   C. 1 week
   D. 5 days
   E. 3 days

459. When tolmetin is used it may produce a false-positive test for
   A. glucose
   B. proteinuria
   C. cholininemia
   D. hemoglobinemia
   E. uric acid

460. Most diarrhea remedies contain
   A. kaolin
   B. benzocaine
   C. aluminum oxide
   D. paregoric
   E. citric acid or citrates

461. Another name for methadone is
   A. aminomone
   B. dionin
   C. metaphenone
   D. Dolophine
   E. dolamine

462. Hydroxychloraquine (Plaquenil) should be used only with extreme caution in patients
   A. with heart ailments
   B. that are hypertensive
   C. with burns
   D. that are elderly
   E. with psoriasis

463. Disclosing solutions are used to
   A. stain plaque
   B. act as abrasives
   C. dissolve food particles
   D. wash away food debris
   E. sterilize the oral cavity

464. Which of the following is NOT a natural alkaloid?
A. Ergotamine
B. Scopolamine
C. Papaverine
D. Lobeline
E. Apomorphine

465. Paraldehyde is potentiated by
A. aspirin
B. cephalosporins
C. disulfiram
D. glucose
E. iron salts

466. Carbidopa is used only
A. in early stages of Parkinson's disease
B. in idiopathic Parkinson's disease
C. in arteriosclerotic Parkinson's disease
D. in combination with levodopa
E. alone

467. Acnomel is usually used to treat
A. burns
B. hemorrhoids
C. diarrhea
D. indigestion
E. acne

468. A test solution for alkaloids used to test for completeness of extraction is
A. silver nitrate
B. gold chloride
C. mercury potassium iodide
D. mercuric oxide
E. hydrogen sulfide

469. A group of agents that interfere significantly with the uptake of guanethidine (Ismelin) are the
A. penicillins
B. mercaptopurines
C. coumarins
D. tricyclic antidepressants
E. narcotic anaglesics

470. Which statement correctly describes the solubility of alkaloids?
    A. Sparingly soluble in water, soluble in dilute acid
    B. Sparingly soluble in water, soluble in nonpolar solvent
    C. Sparingly soluble in water, insoluble in dilute acid
    D. Insoluble in water, insoluble in dilute acid
    E. Insoluble in water, insoluble in nonpolar solvent

471. Barrier creams are quite useful in preventing
    A. drug allergies
    B. poison sumac
    C. food allergies
    D. psoriasis
    E. dry skin

472. Which of the following is a stabilizer in magnesia magma?
    A. Benzoic acid
    B. Citric acid
    C. Oxalic acid
    D. Lactic acid
    E. Mandelic acid

473. The active ingredient in Desenex solution is
    A. salicylic acid
    B. glyceryl triacetate
    C. undecylenic acid
    D. basic fushsin
    E. none of the above

474. Enzactin releases which of the following in the presence of fungus?
    A. Undecylenic acid
    B. Salicylic acid
    C. Acetic acid
    D. Nitric acid
    E. Hydrochloric acid

475. Tinactin contains the antifungal
    A. tolnaftate
    B. glyceryl triacetate
    C. zinc undecylenate
    D. undecylenic acid
    E. none of the above

476. Carbidopa enables the dose of levodopa to be diminished by
A. 10%
B. 20-30%
C. 40-45%
D. 50-60%
E. 80%

477. Wool wax alcohol is
A. cholesterol
B. cetyl alcohol
C. stearyl alcohol
D. myricyl alcohol
E. phytosterol

478. Which of the following is a typical ingredient of antacid preparations?
A. Simethicone
B. Magnesium oxide
C. Magnesium carbonate
D. Calcium carbonate
E. All of the above

479. Netilmycin (Netromycin) is classified as a(an)
A. penicillin
B. cephalosporin
C. tetracycline
D. aminoglycoside
E. antifungal

480. Which of the following is often incompatible with many soft contact lenses?
A. Sodium chloride
B. Benzalkonium chloride
C. Sodium borate
D. EDTA
E. Boric acid

481. Midol is used mainly for
A. menstrual cramps
B. headache
C. arthritic pain
D. athlete's foot
E. psoriasis

482. Which of the following should be classified as a deflocculating agent?
   A. Tween 20
   B. Marasperse
   C. Tween 80
   D. Sodium lauryl sulfate
   E. Carbowax

483. Selsun blue is used mainly as a(an)
   A. skin lotion
   B. shampoo
   C. bath additive
   D. ointment
   E. aerosol

484. Saliva substitutes are used to treat
   A. Vincent's agina
   B. xerophthalmia
   C. xerostomia
   D. zymostomia
   E. sore throats (mild)

485. Insulin injection may be distinguished from protamine zinc injection as
   A. insulin injection is more viscous owing to its higher glycerin content
   B. protamine zinc insulin contains no phenol odor
   C. protamine zinc insulin is colorless while insulin injection is yellowish
   D. insulin injection is acid to litmus while protamine is not
   E. protamine zinc insulin injection is a white suspension while insulin injection is a clear fluid

486. Gly-Oxide provides cleansing effects in the mouth by
   A. releasing oxygen
   B. dissolving plaque on teeth
   C. detergent action
   D. stimulating enzymes
   E. dissolving food particles

487. Carbowax compounds may be classified as
A. isomers
B. tautomers
C. polymers
D. epimers
E. none of the above

Match the following:

A. Ainsworth
B. DuBosc
C. Strong-Cobb
D. Stormer
E. Povan
F. Acacia
G. Emetrol
H. Patterson-Kelly
I. Fitz
J. Freon II

488. Aerosol propellant
489. Gum
490. Cyanine dye
491. Carbohydrate mixture
492. Viscosimeter
493. Balance
494. Colorimeter
495. Tablet hardness tester
496. Blender
497. Mill

498. Most depilatories contain
A. thioglycollates
B. bismuth salts
C. sulfur
D. salcylic acid
E. formates

499. The amount of 190 proof required to make 500 cc of 70% alcohol is
    A. 350 cc
    B. 520 cc
    C. 184 cc
    D. 368 cc
    E. 37 cc

500. Which one of the following is insoluble in alcohol?
    A. Resins
    B. Esters
    C. Volatile oils
    D. Ether
    E. Gums

501. What is the pH of a solution which has a hydroxyl ion concentration of 1.0×10^{-11}?
    A. 10
    B. 4
    C. 2
    D. 3
    E. 11

Match the following:

A. Rheology
B. Buffers
C. Tableting
D. Isotonic solutions
E. Emulsions

502. Continental method
503. Granulation
504. Freezing-point depression method
505. Van Slyke equation
506. Newtonian

Match each generic name with the appropriate trade name:

A. Cytadren
B. Tegretol
C. Decadron
D. Fulvicin P/G
E. Synthroid
F. Lopid
G. Talwin
H. Atarax
I. Intal
J. Neo-Synephrine

507. Carbamazepine
508. Cromolyn sodium
509. Gemfibrozil
510. Phenylephrine
511. Levothyroxine
512. Aminoglutethimide
513. Dexamethasone
514. Griseofulvin ultramicrosize
515. Pentazocine
516. Hydroxyzine

517. Trilafon (perphenzine) is used primarily to treat
A. petit mal epilepsy
B. parkinsonism
C. myasthenia gravis
D. coronary insufficiency
E. psychotic disorders

518. Betadine contains
A. benzocaine
B. surfacaine
C. povidone-iodine complex
D. gentian violet
E. betamethionine

519. Which of the following dose forms is specifically covered by the federal Hazardous Substances Labeling Act?
A. Parenterals
B. Aerosols
C. Tinctures
D. Ophthalmic solutions
E. Nitroglycerin tablets

520. The USP specification of a "cool place" includes the range
A. 8 to 15°C
B. 0 to 10°C
C. 0 to 20°C
D. -5 to +5°C
E. none of the above

521. How many cubic centimeters of 1:1000 epinephrine solution are necessary to make 30 cc of 1:5000 solution?
A. 10 cc
B. 6 cc
C. 15 cc
D. 60 cc
E. 8 cc

522. Which of the following antidepressants is also used as an antihypertensive agent?
A. Amitriptyline
B. Iproniazid
C. Paragyline
D. Imipramine
E. Doxepin

523. Solganal (aurothioglucose) is used in the treatment of
A. carcinomas
B. hypothyroidism
C. vascular headaches
D. rheumatoid arthritis
E. tic doloreux

524. Which of the following is not a phenothiazine anti-psychotic?
A. Chlorpromazine (Thorazine)
B. Triflupromazine (Vesprin)
C. Prochlorperazine (Compazine)
D. Promazine (Sparine)
E. Loxapine (Loxitane)

525. Benzocaine is most effective topically in concentrations of
A. 20%
B. 5%
C. 2%
D. 1%
E. 50%

526. Sorbitol is useful mainly as a(an)
A. solubilizer
B. surfactant
C. emulsiffer
D. counterirritant
E. humectant

527. Which of the following ions plays a significant role in preventing convulsions?
A. Potassium
B. Lithium
C. Magnesium
D. Sodium
E. Fluoride

528. Systemic proteolytic enzymes should NEVER be used concomitantly with
A. aspirin
B. anticoagulants
C. muscle relaxants
D. narcotics
E. diuretics

529. Which of the following is useful in severe cases of dysentery?
A. Pyrvinium salts
B. Emetine
C. Lithium salts
D. Praziquantel
E. Sulfamylol

530. A group of substances used as suppository bases that dissolve rather than melt are
A. esters
B. saturated acids
C. carbowaxes
D. unsaturated fatty acids
E. none of the above

531. A sulfa drug that is widely used to treat ophthalmic infections is
A. sulfadiazine
B. sulfapyridole
C. sulfasuxidine
D. sulfapyramidine
E. sulfacetamide

532. Glyoxide is used frequently to treat
A. hypoxia
B. trench mouth
C. worm infestations
D. dental caries
E. dyspepsia

533. Reciprocity of pharmacy licensure is primarily a function of
A. APhA
B. AACP
C. NABP
D. AIHP
E. AFPE

534. Records relating to DEA drugs must be preserved
A. 1 year
B. 2 years
C. 5 years
D. 7 years
E. permanently

535. An agent commonly combined with local anesthetics is
A. epinephrine
B. phenylephrine
C. ephedrine
D. isoproterenol
E. none of the above

536. A patient taking Pyridium should be warned about
A. marked drowsiness
B. gastric distress
C. headaches
D. discoloration of the urine
E. dizziness

537. When nonpolar substances are dissolved in a polar solvent using surfactants, the process is called
A. HLB
B. solubilization
C. emulsification
D. gelatination
E. none of the above

538. Polysorbate is a synonym for
A. spans
B. sodium lauryl sulfate
C. tweens
D. Brij
E. stannous fluoride

539. The antidote for DDT poisoning is
A. adrenalin
B. atropine
C. barbiturate
D. amphetamine
E. glycerol nonacetate

540. Oxycel is used mainly as a(an)
A. thickener
B. emulsifier
C. oxidizing agent
D. hemostatic agent
E. surfactant

541. Crotamiton (Eurax) is used primarily to treat
   A. scabies
   B. hypertension
   C. severe burns
   D. hookworms
   E. photosensitization

542. Which of the following is a class I controlled drug?
   A. Paregoric
   B. Heroin
   C. Morphine
   D. Demerol
   E. None of the above

543. The chemical substance used commonly in running a GI series is
   A. barium sulfate
   B. fluorescein dye
   C. radioactive iodine
   D. sodium bicarbonate
   E. sodium carbonate

544. Colleges of pharmacy are accredited by
   A. AFPE
   B. AACP
   C. ACPE
   D. NABP
   E. none of the above

Match each diagnostic product with the substance it detects:

   A. Occult blood
   B. Blood urea nitrogen
   C. Leukocytes
   D. Urine glucose
   E. Glucose and protein
   F. Bilirubin

545. Clinitest tablets
546. Azostix
547. Hematest
548. Chemstrip L
549. Uristix
550. Ictotest

2. PHARMACOLOGY

DIRECTIONS: For each of the following multiple choice and matching questions, choose the one most appropriate answer.

---

551. The emetic action of morphine is due to
    - A. irritation of gastrointestinal tract
    - B. stimulation of cerebral cortex
    - C. stimulation of medullary vomiting center
    - D. stimulation of emetic chemoreceptor trigger zone
    - E. none of the above

552 One specific side effect of Tridione administration is
    - A. severe gingival hyperplasia
    - B. the glare phenomenon
    - C. respiratory depression
    - D. cerebral depression
    - E. all of the above

553. Colchicine is used mainly to treat
    - A. gout
    - B. arthritis
    - C. diabetes
    - D. carcinomas
    - E. high blood pressure

554. One procedure in the treatment of digitalis intoxication is to
   A. give K+ salts
   B. stop the administration of the drug
   C. administer quinidine
   D. use permanganate or tannin chemical antidote
   E. administer diuretics to the patient

555. The action of quinidine differs from that of digitalis in
   A. decreasing irritability of cardiac muscle
   B. preventing passage of impulses to the ventricle
   C. increasing irritability of heart muscle
   D. reducing conductivity
   E. none of the above

556. Which of the following would be contraindicated during Antabuse therapy?
   A. Pentobarbital
   B. Paraldehyde
   C. Chloral hydrate
   D. Paradione
   E. None of the above

557. A drug administered by inhalation of powder as a prophylactic for asthma is
   A. ephedrine
   B. disodium cromolyn
   C isoproterenol
   D. oxytriphylline
   E. epinephrine

558. Morphine stimulates
   A. biliary and pancreatic secretions
   B. nonpropulsive rhythmic contractions of small intestine of man
   C. propulsive contractions in small intestine of man
   D. propulsive peristaltic waves in colon
   E. human uterus at full term

Match each drug with its principal use:

A. Bronchodilator
B. Diuretic
C. Treatment of shock
D. Antiarrhythmic
E. Antineoplastic

559. Metariminol (Aramide)
560. Ephedrine
561. Cyclothiazide (Anhydron)
562. Bumetanide (Bumex)
563. Bretylium tosylate (Bretylol)

Match each drug with its use:

A. Antiinflammatory
B. Antinauseant
C. Antiarrhythmic
D. Antidote
E. Topical antifungal

564. Verapamil
565. Diphenidol
566. Clotrimazole
567. EDTA
568. Naprosyn

569. N-acetylcysteine is classified as a(an)
A. analgesic
B. antitussive
C. mucolytic agent
D. antitubercular agent
E. protein hydrolysate

570. Drugs used to treat cystic fibrosis include all of the following EXCEPT
A. anticholinergics
B. antibiotics
C. mucolytic agents
D. expectorants
E. pancreatic enzymes

571. Procarbazine (Matulane) is used primarily to treat
   A. ovarian carcinoma
   B. psoriasis
   C. breast carcinoma
   D. melanoma
   E. Hodgkin's disease

572. Overuse of digitalis may result in
   A. habituation
   B. tolerance
   C. addiction
   D. physical dependence
   E. cumulative poisoning

Match the following:

   A. Skeletal muscle relaxant
   B. Megaloblastic anemias
   C. Used in hypertension
   D. Used in arthritis
   E. Nonmercurial diuretic

573. Motrin
574. Curare
575. Furosemide
576. Folic acid
577. Serpasil

578. The brain-stem centers affected most strongly by barbiturates are the
   A. respiratory centers
   B. vasomotor centers
   C. cardioinhibitory centers
   D. cardioacceleratory centers
   E. none of the above

579. The hypnotic dose of a barbiturate
   A. acts mainly on the cerebral cortex
   B. acts primarily on the brain stem
   C. acts primarily on the thalamus
   D. has a general action on the entire central nervous system
   E. none of the above

580. Strychnine deaths in humans usually occur from
   A. cardiac failure
   B. exhaustion of the respiratory center
   C. fatigue of spinal reflexes
   D. fatigue of respiratory muscles
   E. kidney failure

Match the following:

   A. Antiinflammatory
   B. Shock
   C. Coronary dilator
   D. Antimigraine
   E. Antihistaminic

581. Cafergot
582. Amyl nitrite
583. Levophed
584. Ananase
585. Tacaryl

586. Strychnine acts by
   A. stimulating acetylcholine production
   B. stimulating nerve cell metabolism
   C. depressing inhibitory centers in the spinal cord
   D. inhibiting cholinesterase
   E. stimulating production of cholinesterase

587. Aminocaproic acid is used mainly as a(an)
   A. antiepileptic
   B. antihistaminic
   C. systemic hemostatic
   D. blood expander
   E. muscle relaxant

588. The action of digitalis is enhanced by
   A. sodium
   B. calcium
   C. magnesium
   D. potassium
   E. chloride

589. Which of the following may precipitate an asthma attack?
   A. Respiratory acidosis
   B. Viral and bacterial infections
   C. Respiratory alkalosis
   D. Cranberry juice
   E. Chocolate or Coca Cola

590. Dosage of anticonvulsants is adjusted
   A. when attacks occur frequently
   B. every two weeks
   C. every two years
   D. only when side effects are seen
   E. seasonally

591. The first toxic symptoms of digitalis poisoning are
   A. gastrointestinal irritation
   B. undue depression of heart rate
   C. flushing of skin
   D. cerebral excitement
   E. colored vision

592. Enzymatic oxidation of trapped iodides is blocked in the thyroid gland by
   A. iodides
   B. telepaque
   C. thiouracils
   D. penicillin
   E. thyroxin

593. A drug that produces increased contraction of the sphincter iridis by local application is a
   A. parasympathimimetic drug
   B. parasympatholytic drug
   C. sympathomimetic drug
   D. sympatholytic drug
   E. none of the above

Give the chief use of each of the following:

A. Migraine headache
B. Tranquilizer
C. Diuretic
D. Antihistaminic
E. Anticarcinogenic

594. Naqua
595. Velban
596. Librium
597. Cafergot
598. Equanil
599. Diuril
600. Benadryl

Match the following side effects with the drug producing them:

A. Tinnitis
B. Skin rashes
C. Hypertrophy of the gums
D. Discoloration of teeth

601. Soma
602. Dilantin
603. Achromycin
604. Streptomycin

605. Which of the following symptoms is NOT present in digitalis intoxication?
A. AV block
B. Ventricular tachycardia
C. Vomiting
D. Vagal arrest of the heart
E. Visual disturbances

606. Terbutaline has a preference for stimulation of which of the following receptors?
A. Alpha
B. Gamma
C. Beta 1
D. Beta 2
E. Dopaminergic

607. BAL (British Anti-Lewisite) is used to counter the toxic effects of
A. atropine
B. mercury
C. morphine
D. barbiturates
E. digitalis

608. Streptomycin can cause
A. fourth cranial nerve damage
B. eighth cranial nerve damage
C. tenth cranial nerve damage
D. sixth cranial nerve damage
E. blindness

609. Hyperstat IV (diazoxide) is used mainly in treating
A. severe shock
B. diabetic coma
C. emergency reduction of blood pressure
D. massive hemorrhage
E. paralysis agitans

610. Which of the following should NOT be administered to a patient with myasthenia gravis?
A. Prostigmine
B. Digitalis
C. Atropine
D. Curare
E. Insulin

611. Alcohol in the body is
A. oxidized to CO_2 and water
B. excreted mainly by lungs
C. excreted by kidneys
D. excreted by large intestine
E. detoxified bv kidney

612. Which of the following drugs can be used to treat both constipation and diarrhea?
A. Kaopectate
B. Parepectolin
C. Metamucil
D. Polycarbophil
E. Phenophthalein

613. Methanol may cause
A. deafness
B. tetany
C. delirium tremens
D. gastritis
E. blindness

614. The toxicity of methanol is due to its conversion in the body to
A. acetaldehyde
B. formic acid and formaldehyde
C. ethyl alcohol
D. carbonic acid
E. methane

615. Mithramycin (Mithracin) is used primarily to treat
A. resistant staphylococcal infections
B. thyphoid fever
C. testicular tumors
D. breast carcinoma
E. Hodgkin's disease

616. Which of the following may increase the insulin need of diabetics?
A Isoniazid
B Penicillin
C. Glyceryl guaiacolate
D. Aspirin
E. Prednisone

617. Which of the following is NOT significantly absorbed orally?
A. Isoproterenol
B. Cromolyn
C. Ephedrine
D. Caphalexin
E. Theophylline

618. Because the action of dicumarol persists for several days, its continued use may lead to cumulative poisoning which can be counteracted with
A. thrombin
B. protamine sulfate
C. vitamin K
D. gamma globulin
E. heparin

619. Which of the following agents is most useful for carcinoma of the liver?
A. Vinblastine
B. Floxuridine (FUDR)
C. Vincristine
D. Cytarabine (Cytosar)
E. Mercaptopurine

620. Alternate-day steroid therapy is most useful in treating
A. ulcers
B. carcinoma of the lung
C. insulin shock
D. asthma
E corneal ulcers

621. One of epinephrine's actions on the heart is
A. acceleration due to depression of the vagus
B. increase in refractory period
C. depression of the SA node
D. increase in the concentration of the enzyme phosphorylase A
E. none of the above

622. Epinephrine HCl has little or no effect on
A. unbroken skin
B. conjunctiva
C. precapillary sphincter
D. nasal mucosa
E. pupil

623. Epinephrine HCl is used intravenously in a concentration of
   A. 1:100
   B. 1:1000
   C. 2%
   D. 5%
   E. 10%

624. Epinephrine is often included in the administration of local anesthetics because it
   A. enhances analgesic effect
   B. neutralizes irritant action
   C. delays diffusion of the anesthetic from the site of injection
   D. increases diffusion of the anesthetic
   E. increases blood levels of the anesthetic

625. Tromethamine is used to prevent
   A. rickets
   B. dental caries
   C. spontaneous abortion
   D. infections
   E. acidosis

626. Rafampin may do all of the following EXCEPT
   A. decrease BUN and serum uric acid
   B. cause teratogenic effects
   C. produce liver dysfunction
   D. color urine and feces
   E. inhibit effect of oral contraceptives

627. Which type of patient is most likely to be hypersensitive to aspirin?
   A. Intrinsic asthmatic
   B. Extrinsic asthmatic
   C. Chronic bronchitic
   D. Patient with viral infection
   E. C and D

628. The principal active alkaloid of ipecac is
   A. yohimbine
   B. caffeine
   C. apomorphine
   D. lobeline
   E. emetine

629. Emetine is used in the treatment of
   A. malaria
   B. schistosomiasis
   C. tuberculosis
   D. amebiasis
   E. none of the above

630. Sensitization of the heart to epinephrine is a possible danger in the use of
   A. cyclopropane
   B. nitrous oxide
   C. ether
   D. vinyl ether
   E. pentotothal

631 The therapeutic use of neostigmine bromide is as a
   A. miotic
   B. CNS depressant
   C. treatment of curare poisoning
   D. neuromuscular blocker
   E. muscle relaxant

632. Ethylenediamine-tetraacetic acid is an antidote for which of the following?
   A. Sodium secobarbital
   B. Aspirin
   C. Paris green
   D. Phosphorus
   E. Lead

633. Which of the following drugs requires repeated prothrombin time determinations during its administration?
   A. Heparin
   B. Dicumarol
   C. Quinidine
   D. Protamine
   E. Regitine

634. The antispasmodic action of papaverine on smooth muscle is exerted
  A. via stimulation of parasympathetic ganglia in intestinal wall
  B. via stimulation of sympathetic ganglia in intestinal wall
  C. directly on muscle cell
  D. through central nervous system
  E. by parasympathetic blocking action

635. Naquical is a product which contains a combination of
  A. digoxin and hydrochlorothiazine
  B. spironolactone and reserpine
  C. urea and gitalin
  D. chlorothiazide and hydrochlorothiazide
  E. trichlormethiazide and reserpine

636. Side effects due to administration of ganglionic blocking drugs for the treatment of hypertension do NOT include
  A. constipation
  B. urinary retention
  C. impairment of visual accommodation
  D. profuse sweating
  E. dryness of mouth

637. Paxipam (halazepam) is used primarily to treat
  A. edema
  B. congestive heart failure
  C. symptoms of anxiety
  D. epilepsy
  E. muscle spasms

638. Isoetharine is a drug which stimulates primarily which of the following receptors?
  A. Alpha
  B. Histamine
  C. Beta 1
  D. Beta 2
  E. None of the above

639. Large doses of diethylstilbestrol are used to treat carcinoma of the
   A. vaginal tract
   B. bone marrow
   C. liver
   D. kidney
   E. prostate

640. The primary use of methocyflurane is as a(an)
   A. anesthetic
   B. analgesic
   C. cardiac stimulant
   D. hypnotic
   E. hypotensive agent

641. In case of acute pain of angina pectoris the most effective treatment would be to administer
   A. mannitol hexanitrate
   B. erythrityl tetranitrate
   C. sodium nitrate
   D. pentaerythritol tetranitrate
   E. nitroglycerin

642. The mechanism explaining the clinical picture observed in carbon monoxide poisoning is
   A. hemolysis of red blood cells
   B. a chemical union of the carbon monoxide with the hemoglobin of the red blood cells
   C. transformation of the carbon monoxide to carbon dioxide in the blood
   D. arrest of oxidation in the tissues by enzyme interference
   E. none of the above

643. Chloramphenicol is particulary effective in the treatment of
   A. diphtheria
   B. tuberculosis
   C. emphysema
   D. rickettsial diseases
   E. Streptomyces pyogenes infections

644. An advantage of bleomycin over most antineoplastic drugs is its
A. rapid onset of action
B. lack of toxicity to all normal cells
C. relative lack of bone marrow toxicity
D. very broad spectrum of activity
E. A and B

645. Heparin therapy is best controlled with
A. prothrombin time
B. platelet counts
C. bleeding times
D. clotting times
E. no controls are needed

646. Pilocarpine would produce which of the following?
A. Constriction of pupil of the eye
B. Mydriasis
C. Cycloplegia
D. Tachycardia
E. None of the above

647. The drug of choice for scarlet fever is
A. tetracycline
B. sulfonamides
C. penicillin
D. chloromycetin
E. novobiocin

648. The major action of Proventil (albuterol) is
A. diuretic activity
B. vasoconstriction
C. anticholinergic
D. peripheral vasodilation
E. bronchodilation

649. Acetylcholine has both muscarinic and nicotinic actions. The muscarinic action can be blocked by
A. epinephrine
B. atropine
C. nicotine
D. curare
E. nicotine and curare

650. Which of the following is NOT an estrogenic substance?
    A. Estradiol
    B. Premarin
    C. Theelin
    D. Follicle-stimulating hormone
    E. Stilbesterol

651. Sulfonamides are excreted free and combined as the
    A. acetyl derivative
    B. amino derivative
    C. sulfate derivative
    D. glycine conjugate
    E. none of the above

652. Glucagon is used as a substitute for anticholinergics in radiological examination of the
    A. liver
    B. kidney
    C. spleen
    D. GI tract
    E. bone marrow

653. An antifungal that releases acetic acid only in the presence of fungus is
    A. Enzactin
    B. Desenex
    C. Vioform
    D. Grisactin
    E. Mycostatin

654. Which of the following is the fastest acting anticoagulant?
    A. Warfarin (Coumadin)
    B. Heparin
    C. Ouabain
    D. Protamine sulfate
    E. Vitamin K

655. An advantage of ephedrine sulfate over epinephrine is that it
A. is nontoxic
B. is more potent
C. is effective orally
D. decreases skeletal muscle tone
E. is more soluble

656. Meperidine produces analgesia equal to that of morphine in a dose how many times that of morphine?
A. 1/2
B. 8-10
C. Equal
D. 100
E. 1/10

657. Which of the following is a gametocidal agent in malaria?
A. Atabrine
B. Quinine
C. Paludrine
D. Primaquine
E. Aralen

658. Gyne-Lotrimin (clotrimazole) is effective in treating
A. amenorrhea
B. spontaneous abortion
C. dysmenorrhea
D. moniliasis
E. postpartum bleeding

659. Excessive use of tolbutamide will lead to
A. diarrhea
B. prolonged hypoglycemia
C. tolerance to alcohol
D. acidosis
E. glycosuria

660. Which of the following is contraindicated in the presence of active tuberculosis?
A. Hydrocortisone
B. Streptomycin
C. INH
D. PAS
E. PABA

661. Which of the following would be the drug of choice for treatment of hypertensive crisis?
A. Diazoxide (Hyperstat)
B. Clonidine (Catapres)
C. Propranolol (Inderal)
D. Guanethidine (Ismelin)
E. Reserpine (Serpasil)

662. The major disadvantage in the use of meperidine is that it produces
A. low blood pressure
B. high blood pressure
C. addiction
D. miosis
E. severe respiratory depression

663. Parkinsonism is probably due to
A. too little dopamine in the brain
B. too little levodopa in the brain
C. too little acetylcholine in the brain
D. too much levodopa in the brain
E. too much dopamine in the brain

664. A group of agents used primarily for breast carcinomas are
A. androgens
B. estrogens
C. ethylaminobenzoates
D. digitalis glycosides
E. veratrum alkaloids

665. An overdose of d-tubocurarine
A. interferes with oxidative enzymes of the cells
B. paralyzes respiratory muscles
C. may be combatted with carbachol
D. paralyzes the autonomic nervous system
E. depresses the medullary respiratory center

666. All antihistamines appear to antagonize histamine by
A. blocking release of histamine from mast cells
B. histaminase action
C. blocking synthesis of histamine
D. competing with histamine for cell receptors
E. none of the above

667. Codeine acts as a cough sedative by
A. producing mild nausea
B. depressing bronchiolar secretions
C. depressing pulmonary action
D. depressing cough center
E. paralyzing sensory nerves of bronchi

668. Organic pesticides may be effectively counteracted with
A. pentazocine
B. dopamine
C. neutrapen
D. pralidoxime
E. charcoal

669. Patients receiving iron therapy should be warned about
A. dizziness
B. ringing in the ears
C. danger of sunlight
D. blackening of the stool
E. paresthesia

670. Phenothiazines are not effective in control of vomiting due to
A. radiation
B. infection
C. digitalis
D. upset stomach
E. motion sickness

671. The greatest threat from morphine poisoning is
A. renal shutdown
B. paralysis of spinal cord
C. respiratory depression
D. cardiovascular collapse
E. none of the above

672. Negatol (Negatan) is used primarily to control
   A. arterial bleeding
   B. venous bleeding
   C. large vessel bleeding
   D. capillary bleeding
   E. surgical bleeding

673. Which of the following is a direct-acting vasodilator used to treat hypertension?
   A. Amyl nitrite
   B. Clonidine (Catapres)
   C. Methyldopa (Aldomet)
   D. Pargyline (Eutonyl)
   E. Prazosin (Minipress)

674. An advantage of betamethasone acetate over betamethasone sodium phosphate is
   A. fewer allergic reactions
   B. prompter action
   C. more sustained action
   D. greater solubility
   E. there is no advantage

675. A specific narcotic antagonist is
   A. meperidine
   B. polybrene
   C. nalorphine
   D. universal antidote
   E. meprobamate

676. Ritodrine (Yutapar) is used to control
   A. diarrhea
   B. dyspnea
   C. pernicious anemia
   D. preterm labor
   E. convulsions

677. A very common side effect of morphine is
   A. allergic response
   B. blood dyscrasias
   C. constipation
   D. liver damage
   E. visceral pain

678. Which of the following is used to curtail chronic uric-acid stone formation?
   A. Allopurinol
   B. Trimethoprim
   C. Methenamine
   D. Ethacrynic acid
   E. Furosemide

679. Which of the following drugs is a monamine oxidase inhibitor, but is used to treat hypertension?
   A. Tranylcypromine (Parnate)
   B. Reserpine
   C. Propranolol (Inderal)
   D. Pargyline (Eutonyl)
   E. Imipramine (Tofranil)

680. A prominent toxic effect of local anesthetics is
   A. CNS stimulation
   B. CNS depression
   C. tachycardia
   D. local ischemia
   E. none of the above

681. Among the signs of barbiturate poisoning are
   A. hypertension
   B. diuresis
   C. decreased respiratory volume
   D. alkalosis
   E. none of the above

682. A drug that is very effective in the treatment of tinea versicolor is
   A. undecylenic acid
   B. clotrimazole (Lotrimin)
   C. acrisorcin (Akrinol)
   D. penicillin G
   E. prednisolone

683. Which of the following is characteristic of vasopressin?
   A. Antidiuretic effect
   B. Constricts capillaries
   C. Coronary vasoconstriction
   D. Increased motility of bowel
   E. All of the above

684. A potent tranquilizer which also exhibits strong hypotensive effects is
A. Librium
B. meprobamate
C. reserpine
D. Thorazine
E. Sparine

685. Which of the following is used to lower blood lipid levels?
A. Trimethadione
B. Clofibrate
C. Flucytosine
D. Coumarin
E. Propranolol

686. Which of the following is a first-line drug to treat tuberculosis?
A. PAS
B. Rifampin
C. Ethionamide
D. Cycloserine
E. Ethambutol

Match each group of drugs with its site of action:

A. Subcortical levels of CNS
B. Dopamine receptors
C. Medulla
D. Parietal cells
E. Small and large colon

687. Histamine antagonists for ulcer treatment
688. Opium alkaloids for treatment of cough
689. Benzodiazepines
690. Bulk producers
691. Phenothiazines

Match each drug with its mechanism of action:

A. Slows intestinal motility
B. Neuromuscular blockade
C. Inhibits release of norepinephrine
D. Converts to depamine in brain
E. Blocks decarboxylation in peripheral circulation

692. Carbidopa
693. L-Dopa
694. Vercuronium (Norcuron)
695. Guanethidine (Ismelin)
696. Loperomide HCl (Imodium)

Match the following pharmacological actions with the drug which will produce the effect:

A. Cimetidine
B. Sinequan
C. Dantrium
D. Dymelor
E. Parepectolin

697. Antidiarrheal action
698. Muscle relaxation
699. Mood elevation
700. Lowering of blood sugar
701. Inhibits actions of histamine

Match each drug with its prevalent adverse effect:

A. Light-headedness
B. Severe gastric upset
C. Tinnitis
D. Anaphylaxis
E. Skin eruptions

702. Indocin
703. Gantrisin
704. Penicillin G
705. Sinutabs
706. Quinidine

707. Which of the following could be used as an antidote for curare poisoning?
   A. Neostigmine
   B. Atropine
   C. Homatropine
   D. Hexamethonium
   E. None of the above

Match the following:

   A. Very low toxicity
   B. Has action on striated muscle
   C. Produces severe GI symptoms
   D. Acridine dye which causes yellowing of skin
   E. Has adverse effects on the black race

708. Quinine
709. Quinacrine
710. Primaquine
711. Chloroquine
712. Daraprim

   A. Useful for induction in patients with broncho-constriction
   B. Tachypnea is a sign of overdosage
   C. Will not produce adequate muscular relaxation
   D. Gas with 100% potency
   E. Relatively impotent and explosive

713. Trichloroethylene
714. Nitrous oxide
715. Cyclopropane
716. Ethylene
717. Divinyl ether

Match the following:

A. Ultra short-acting barbiturate
B. Short-acting barbiturate
C. Intermediate-acting barbiturate
D. Long-acting barbiturate
E. Nonbarbiturate

718. Chloral hydrate
719. Phenobarbital
720. Amobarbital
721. Secobarbital
722. Thiopental

Match each drug or drug group with a specific contra-indication:

A. Adrenal insufficiency
B. Bronchopulmonary disease
C. Thrombophlebitis
D. Blood dyscrasias
E. Pregnancy

723. Oral contraceptives
724. Trilostane (Modrastone)
725. Probenicid
726. Ergotamine derivatives
727. Paraldehyde

728. Therapeutically vitamin B_1 has been employed most usccessfully in the treatment of
A. microcytic anemia
B. pellagra
C. scurvy
D. beriberi
E. macrocytic anemia

729. Aminophylline is used most frequently in
A. asthma
B. nephritic edema
C. lowering cerebral pressure
D. eliminating toxins in the body
E. diabetes insipidus

730. Propylthiouracil is useful in the treatment of
   A. derangement toxicosis
   B. hypothyroidism
   C. hypoparathyroidism
   D. hyperthyroidism
   E. thyroiditis

731. A serious side effect of Alkeran is
   A. phagocytosis
   B. tolerance develops rapidly
   C. depression of WBC
   D. severe kidney damage
   E. visual disturbances

Match the following drugs with the most closely related statement:

   A. An anticoagulant which interferes with prothrombin synthesis
   B. An antihistamine
   C. Used to control postpartum bleeding
   D. An anthelminthic
   E. A nucleic acid antimetabolite

732. Ergonovine
733. Thiabendazole
734. 6-Mercaptopurine
735. Bishydroxycoumarin
736. Brompheniramine

Match each drug with a major drug interaction:

   A. Propoxyphene
   B. Theophylline
   C. Acidifying agents
   D. Potassium ion
   E. Isoniazid

737. Phenytoin
738. Carbamazepine
739. Colchicine
740. Diazepam
741. Pancuronium

742. Yellow pigmentation of the skin is most common with
- A. chloraquine
- B. pamaquin
- C. quinacrine
- D. quinine
- E. atabrine

Match the following:

- A. Used in treatment of addiction
- B. Analgesic with some antispasmodic action
- C. Most abundant alkaloid in opium
- D. Weakest of the phenanthrene analgesics
- E. No antagonism by nalorphine

743. Codeine
744. Papaverine
745. Meperidine
746. Methadone
747. Morphine

748. Meticorten (prednisone) is classified as a(an)
- A. antifungal
- B. analgesic
- C. muscle relaxant
- D. antihistaminic
- E. antiinflammatory

Match the following:

- A. Muscle relaxant
- B. Antifungal
- C. Analgesic
- D. Diuretic
- E. Miotic

749. Dyazide
750. Florinal
751. Tinactin
752. Physostigmine
753. Valium

754. Cigarette smoking increases the side effects of
A. narcotic analgesics
B. analeptics
C. antidepressants
D. oral contraceptives
E. cardiac glycosides

755. Spironolactone acts by antagonizing
A. insulin
B. glucagon
C. aldosterone
D. histamine
E. A and C

756. Which of the following does NOT represent an action of quinidine on the myocardium?
A. Increases the refractory period
B. Increases force of contraction of the muscle
C. Raises the fibrillation threshold
D. Blocks vagal effects on heart
E. Slows conduction

757. Which of the following does NOT enhance the potential effects of digitalis on the heart?
A. Increased renal clearance
B. Myocardial anoxia
C. Alkalosis
D. Low serum potassium
E. High serum calcium

758. Which of the following groups antagonizes the activity of guanethidine (Ismelin) in treating hypertension?
A. Narcotic analgesics
B. Thiazides
C. Sulfonamides
D. Phenothiazines
E. Osmotic diuretics

759. Vivactil (protriptyline) is used mainly as a(an)
A. analgesic
B. muscle relaxant
C. cardiotonic
D. antidepressant
E. antispasmodic

760. Which of the following commonly stimulates the emetic mechanism as a prevalent side effect?
A. Unitensin
B. Minipress
C. Inderal
D. Aldomet
E. Ismelin

Match each drug with the pharmacological class to which it belongs:

A. Calcium channel blocker
B. Emetic
C. Antivertigo agent
D. Analgesic
E. GI antispasmodic

761. Dicyclomine (Bentyl)
762. Diphenidol (Vontrol)
763. Verapamil HCl (Calan)
764. Apomorphine HCl
765. Methotrimeprazine

766. Which is the drug of choice for trigeminal neuralgia?
A. Carbamazepine
B. Phenytoin
C. Flurazepam
D. Diazepam
E. Trimethadione

767. The most effective drug for prophylaxis against meningitis is
A. penicillin G
B penicillin V
C. tetracycline
D. erythromycin
E. sulfisoxazole

768. Which of the following may increase seizure activity in epileptic patients?
A. Ethotoin
B. Phenobarbital
C. Trihexyphenidyl
D. Amantadine
E. L-Dopa

769. Cimetadine (Tagamet) is used to treat
   A. hypertension
   B. muscular injuries
   C. ulcers
   D. edema
   E. congestive heart failure

770. Magnesium ion is necessary in
   A. stimulating enzyme systems
   B. muscular contraction
   C. nerve conduction
   D. all of the above
   E. none of the above

771. Which of the following diuretics does NOT cause appreciable muscular weakness or cramping?
   A. Amiloride (Colectril)
   B. Ethacrynic acid (Edecrin)
   C. Polythiazide (Renese)
   D. Cyclothiazide (Anhydron)
   E. Methyclothiazide (Enduron)

772. Trazodone (Desyrel) is used primarily as a(an)
   A. analgesic
   B. cardiotonic
   C. tranquilizer
   D. antidepressant
   E. antihypertensive

773. Vitamin A and D ointment is useful in treating
   A. rickets
   B. avitaminosis
   C. puncture wounds
   D. minor burns and skin irritation
   E. tinea infestations

Match each drug with a prevalent side effect:

A. Breakthrough bleeding
B. Nasal dryness
C. Corneal damage
D. Thyroid enlargement
E. Diarrhea

774. DMSO
775. Norethindrone
776. Tolbutamide (Orinase)
777. Ethacrynic acid (Edecrin)
778. Flunisolide (Nasalide)

779. The principal difference between competitive and non-competitive inhibition is
A. extent of receptor site blocking
B. whether inhibition occurs
C. extent of enzyme inhibition
D. degree of agonism
E. none of the above

780. Hypokalemia as a side effect of diuretic therapy can be diminished most safely with
A. citrus fruits
B. salt
C. potassium salts
D. seafood
E. mixed electrolytes

781. In addition to their marked potency, the loop diuretics Lasix and Edecrin have an added advantage of
A. being completely free of side effects
B. causing hypokalemia
C. not causing any electrolyte imbalance
D. requiring only once weekly dosing
E. being effective when given orally

782. A class of plant alkaloids that are widely used to treat migraine are
   A. vinca alkaloids
   B. digitalis glycosides
   C. stramonium alkaloids
   D. ergot alkaloids
   E. belladonna alkaloids

Match the following:

   A. Coronary vasodilator
   B. Antihypertensive
   C. General anesthetic
   D. Appetite suppressant
   E. To treat shock

783. Preludin
784. Nitroglycerin
785. Levophed
786. Ismelin
787. Ether

788. Alcohol hallucinosis is commonly treated with
   A. disulfiram (Antabuse)
   B. phenothiazines
   C. barbiturates
   D. caffeine
   E. oxygen

789. A toxic effect of alcohol is
   A. mitosis
   B. mydriasis
   C. agranulocytosis
   D. CNS stimulation
   E. respiratory depression

790. Which of the following is a serotonin antagonist?
   A. Glutethimide
   B. Caffeine
   C. Tolbutamide
   D. Triplelennamine
   E. Methysergide

791. Bisacodyl frequently can cause
   A. abdominal cramps
   B. constipation
   C. skin rashes
   D. dizziness
   E. nausea

Match each of the following drugs with the condition it most often causes:

A. Agranulocytosis
B. Respiratory alkalosis
C. Toxic cirrhosis of the liver
D. Methemoglobinemia

792. Acetylsalicylic acid
793. Acetanilid
794. Aminopyrine

Match each vitamin with a major role that it plays:

A. Bone formation
B. Hematopoiesis
C. Protein metabolism
D. Assists night vision

795. Vitamin A
796. Vitamin B_6
797. Vitamin B_{12}
798. Vitamin D

Relate the following:

A. Causes involution of thyroid gland with colloid storage
B. Does not prevent iodide uptake
C. Suppresses thyroxin formation and decreases amount of colloid in thyroid gland
D. Stimulates release and synthesis of thyroxin
E. More potent than thyroxin

799. Triiodothyronine
800. Thyrotropic hormone
801. Thiouracil
802. Iodide

Match each drug with its common use:

A. Reduce blood lipids
B. Abortifacient
C. Treat anemias
D. Hypnotic
E. Coronary thrombosis
F. Antihemophilic
G. Treatment of acne
H. Laxative
I. Anticonvulsant

803. Simron
804. Streptokinase
805. Factor IX complex
806. Carboprost
807. Gemfibrozil (Lopid)
808. Methaqualone (Quaalude)
809. Clonazepam (Clonopin)
810. Mucilose
811. Vitamin A acid

Match the statement with the most appropriate drug:

A. Polymyxin
B. Sulfonamides
C. Penicillin
D. Tetracycline
E. Sulfones
F. Isoniazid

812. Inhibited by PABA
813. Skin eruptions are the most common type of allergic response
814. Eradicates both cysts and trophozoites of intestinal amebiasis from the feces
815. Neurotoxic upon parenteral administration
816. Equal or superior to streptomycin as an antitubercular drug
817. Drug of choice for Hansen's disease

Match the following:

A. Enzyme used for leukemia
B. From a plant source
C. Should only be given IV
D. May be incorporated into RNA and DNA
E. Cytotoxic action largely limited to bone marrow

818. Vincristine
819. Asparaginase
820. Myleran
821. 6-Mercaptopurine
822. Mechlorethamine

Match the following disease or condition with the drug used to treat it:

A. Allopurinol
B. Chlorpromazine
C. Tolbutamide
D. Diphenhydramine
E. Diphenylhydantoin
F. Ergotamine
G. Pentobarbital
H. Amphetamines

823. Diabetes
824. Hay fever
825. Nausea
826. Migraine
827. Epilepsy
828. Gout
829. Insomnia
830. Obesity

Match each of the following on the basis of pharmacological similarity:

A. Furosemide
B. Glyburide
C. Cimetidine
D. Hydrochlorethiazide
E. Mefenemic acid
F. Gaviscon
G. Verapamil HCl

831. Ranitidine
832. Idipamide
833. Bumetamide
834. Glipizide
835. Amphojel
836. Zomopirac
837. Nifedipine

838. A common side effect of ephedrine is
A. rashes
B. nervousness
C. blood dyscrasias
D. drowsiness
E. ulcers

839. Titanium dioxide is used primarily in which of the following preparations?
A. Cough
B. Sunscreen
C. Topical anesthetic
D. Topical antiseptic
E. Burn treatment

Match the following drugs to the correct route of metabolism or metabolic product:

A. Side-chain oxidation in liver
B. Trichlorethanol glucuronide
C. Gentisic acid
D. Methyluric acid
E. Methylation of orthodydroxy group
F. 5-OH indoleacetic acid
G. Hydrolysis by plasma cholinesterase
H. Acetylation
I. Sulfoxide formation
J. Excreted via lungs unchanged

840. Salicylates
841. Epinephrine
842. Ether
843. Phenobarbital
844. Serotonin
845. Succinylcholine
846. Sulfonamides
847. Chloral hydrate
848. Caffeine
849. Chlorpromazine

Match each statement with the most appropriate drug:

A. Phenacemid (Phenurone)
B. Diphenylhydantoin (Dilantin)
C. Pentylenetetrazol (Metrazol)
D. Methylphenylethylhydantoin (Mesantoin)
E. Paramethadione (Paradione)
F. Primidone (Mysoline)

850. Effective against grand mal seizures
851. Effective against petit mal seizures
852. One of the most toxic of the clinically available antiepileptics
853. Intensifies the preictal aura
854. Combined use with trimethadione or paramethadione is especially prone to cause severe toxic reactions
855. A central nervous system stimulant

Match the following:

A. Antagonist to norepinephrine
B. Antidote for mercuhydrin
C. Direct action on uterine musculature
D. Inhibits release of norepinephrine from adrenergic nerves
E. Given IV as Ca, Na salt
F. Carbonic anhydrase inhibitor
G. Folic acid antagonist
H. Antidote for cyanide
I. DFP antidote
J. Inhibits oxidation of alcohol at the acetaldehyde stage

856. EDTA
857. Aminopterin
858. BAL
859. Bretylium
860. Sodium nitrite
861. Dibenamine
862. Tetraethylthiuram disulfide
863. Oxytocin
864. Diamox (acetazolamide)
865. Atropine

Match each drug with its prevalent side effect:

A. Constipation
B. Respiratory distress
C. Postural hypotension
D. Stomatitis
E. Agranulocytosis
F. Drowsiness

866. Reserpine
867. Mercurophylline
868. Morphine
869. Thioridazine
870. Dimenhydrinate

Match each drug with a major use:

A. Diuretic
B. Antiarrhythmic
C. Antithyroid drug
D. Antihypertensive
E. Antihyperlipidemic

871. Mannitol
872. Propylthiouracil
873. Bretylium tosylate
874. Minoxidil
875. Clofibrate

876. Thiazide diuretics may produce an increase in blood levels of uric acid and
A. potassium
B. BUN
C. urea
D. lithium
E. glucose

877. An advantage of nortriptyline (Aventyl) over other dibenzazepines is that it
A. has a longer duration of action
B. is far less toxic
C. is more soluble
D. acts faster
E. is usually given parenterally

878. The most effective single chemotherapeutic agent of those indicated, in the treatment of tuberculosis is
A. neomycin
B. sulfones
C. streptomycin
D. penicillin
E. terramycin

879. Eutonyl (pargyline) is specifically contraindicated in
   A. diabetes
   B. hypertension
   C. frostbite
   D. hyperthyroidism
   E. heart failure

880. Which of the following statements is true of heparin?
   A. Obtained from spoiled sweet clover
   B. Destroyed in intestinal tract
   C. Does not prevent clotting of shed blood
   D. Inhibits prothrombin synthesis in liver
   E. None of the above

881. Which of the following statements is true of bishydroxycoumarin?
   A. Obtained from cattle lung
   B. Has antithrombin action
   C. Prevents clotting of shed blood
   D. Not antagonized by fresh whole blood
   E. None of the above

882. Elspar (asparaginase) is used primarily as a(an)
   A. inhibitor of secretions
   B. antipsychotic
   C. hemostatic agent
   D. antineoplastic
   E. coronary vasodilator

883. The chief use of levoarterenol is to treat
   A. shock
   B. diabetes
   C. hypertension
   D. cardiac arrhythmias
   E. iron deficiencies

884. Tolerance to nitroglycerin may be overcome by
   A. initially using the largest safe dose of the drug
   B. using other nitrites
   C. temporarily discontinuing the drug for one or two weeks
   D. use of higher doses
   E. none of the above

885. The site of action of thiazide diuretics is primarily the
A. tubule just beyond the loop of Henle
B. loop of Henle
C. proximal tubule
D. B and C
E. A and C

886. Ethacrynic acid is used primarily as a(an)
A. diuretic
B. antiemetic
C. laxative
D. sedative
E. analgesic

887. Antihistamines have little effect on which of the following actions of histamine?
A. Bronchospasm
B. Wheal and flare
C. Hypotension
D. Gastric secretion
E. Increased capillary permeability

888. Acute bronchial asthma is an indication for all of the following EXCEPT
A. epinephrine
B. ephedrine
C. aminophylline
D. prednisolone
E. bradykinin

889. Parnate exerts its action by
A. producing epinephrine
B. inhibiting acetylcholine
C. inhibiting MAO
D. direct action on medulla
E. direct action on spinal cord

890. An advantage of Dopram over other analeptics is
A. short duration of action
B. long duration of action
C. it does not depress respiration
D. dosage easier to adjust
E. none of the above

891. Which of the following is used to relieve GI muscle spasm?
A. Edrophonium (Tensilon)
B. Bethanechol (Urecholine)
C. Guanethidine (Ismelin)
D. Epinephrine
E. Dicyclomine (Bentyl)

892. Which of the following is used to prevent local necrosis from neoprinephrine infusions?
A. Propranolol (Inderal)
B. Phentolamine (Regitine)
C. Ephedrine
D. Dopamine
E. Edrophonium (Tensilon)

893. Isoxuprine is used to treat
A. asthma
B. severe hypotension
C. nasal congestion
D. premature labor
E. hypertension

894. Which is an antidote for malathion poisoning?
A. Vitamin K
B. Protamine sulfate
C. Nalorphine (Nalline)
D. Pralidoxime (Protopam)
E. Edrophonium (Tensilon)

895. The usual dosage schedule of thiazide diuretics is
A. q 4 h
B. qid
C. tid
D. weekly
E. once daily

896. A group of drugs used widely to treat mild hypertension is
A. sympathetic blockers
B. diuretics
C. ganglionic blockers
D. MAO inhibitors
E. none of the above

897. Pimozide (Orap) should not be used in patients with a history of
   A. asthma
   B. cardiac arrhythmias
   C. drug abuse
   D. alcoholism
   E. allergies

898. Clinoril (Sulindac) is most properly classified as an
   A. antirheumatic
   B. antihypertensive
   C. antipsychotic
   D. antiemetic
   E. antispasmodic

899. What is the advantage of levodopa over dopamine in treating parkinsonism?
   A. It is more stable
   B. It is less toxic
   C. It is more readily available
   D. It is considerably less expensive
   E. It is more effective

900. Cyclosporine is used for
   A. allergies
   B. angina
   C. prevention of transplant rejection
   D. steroid deficiency
   E. treating lead poisoning

3. MICROBIOLOGY AND PUBLIC HEALTH

DIRECTIONS: For each of the following multiple choice and matching questions, choose the one most appropriate answer.

901. Vidarabine is effective against
    A. syphilis
    B. gonorrhea
    C. typhoid fever
    D. herpes simplex
    E. all of the above

902. A useful precaution when administering live virus vaccines is to have available
    A. antiviral agents
    B. plasma expanders
    C. whole blood
    D. glucose solution
    E. epinephrine solution

903. Diagnostic diphtheria toxin
    A. is used in Schick test
    B. contains phenol as a bacteriostatic agent
    C. is injected intradermally in an amount equivalent to 1 MLD dose in a guinea pig
    D. is injected intramuscularly
    E. is 1.0 cc in dose

904. Which of the following is classified as an antiviral agent?
   A. Novobiocin
   B. Gentamicin
   C. Amphotericin B
   D. Rifampin
   E. Vidarabine

905. A most useful antibiotic to treat serious infections caused by Pseudomonas aeruginosa strains is
   A. rifampin
   B. novobiocin
   C. kanamycin
   D. gentamicin
   E. clindamicin

906. Yellow fever vaccine
   A. is a suspension in water for injection
   B. consists of killed strain of yellow fever virus
   C. is a living culture of an attenuated strain of yellow fever virus
   D. requires no special labelling
   E. imparts immunity which lasts for less than 1 year

907. Which of the following groups depresses the activity of griseofulvin?
   A. Barbiturates
   B. Dibenzazepines
   C. Topical antifungals
   D. Diazepoxides
   E. Anticoagulants

Match the following:

   A. Precipitate solutions of bacterial substances
   B. Do not require complement
   C. Require complement for bactericidal action
   D. Are not bactericidal but promote phagocytosis
   E. Antibodies easily destroyed by heat

908. Bacteriolysins
909. Bacteriotropins
910. Opsonins
911. Agglutinins
912. Precipitins

913. Smallpox vaccine
   A. is obtained from vaccinated horses
   B. is prepared by making a glycerol-water suspension of vesicles of vaccinia or cowpox
   C. must be acid to bromocresol purple
   D. is not stable when frozen
   E. is injected intramuscularly

914. Rabies vaccine
   A. may be stored at room temperature
   B. provides permanent immunity
   C. must be tested for noninfectivity in rabbits
   D. is prepared from street virus
   E. is prepared from serum of infected rabbits

915. Rabies virus is attenuated by
   A. drying
   B. dilution
   C. emulsification with phenol
   D. all of the above
   E. none of the above

916. Live vaccines are not used in this country for immunization against
   A. diphtheria
   B. measles
   C. poliomyelitis
   D. rabies
   E. smallpox

917. North American anti-snakebite serum is effective against the bite of
   A. copperhead
   B. cottonmouth moccasin
   C. rattlesnake
   D. all of the above
   E. none of the above

918. Rubella is another name for
   A. measles
   B. meningitis
   C. german measles
   D. scarlet fever
   E. mumps

919. The antitoxic effect of tetanus antitoxin lasts
   A. 4-6 hours
   B. 24 hours
   C. indefinitely
   D. 2-3 years
   E. 10 days

920. If symptoms of tetanus appear, the antitoxin should
   A. be given subcutaneously
   B. be given orally
   C. be given intramuscularly
   D. be given intravenously or intraspinally
   E. not be given

921. Live rubella virus vaccines provide immunization for
   A. 1 year
   B. 3 years
   C. 6 years
   D. 10 years
   E. lifetime

922. Antitoxins are usually associated with which of the following fractions of the blood?
   A. Euglobulin
   B. Pseudoglobulin
   C. Albumin
   D. Leukocyte
   E. Fibrinogen

923. Toxins
   A. are measured in terms of their MLD for a certain laboratory animal
   B. lose combining power with antitoxin before potency
   C. are unstable when dried in vacuo
   D. are unstable even if dried in vacuo and stored at 0°C
   E. none of the above

924. A common complaint after vaccination with live rubella virus vaccine is
   A. rash
   B. sore throat
   C. headache
   D. pain in the joints
   E. polyneuritis

925. Which of the following exerts its effect by interference with cell wall synthesis?
   A. Griseofulvin (Fulvicin)
   B. Nystatin (Mycostatin)
   C. Flucytosine (Ancobon)
   D. Cephalothin (Keflin)
   E. Tolnaftate (Tinactin)

926. Poliomyelitis vaccine
   A is made from type 1 and 2 strains only
   B. should not be used if color changes
   C. may be used if turbid
   D. should not be allowed to freeze and refreeze constantly
   E. contains polio virus killed with cresol

927. Black death is the term associated with
   A. diphtheria
   B. whooping cough
   C. tularemia
   D. brucellosis
   E. sylvatic plague

928. Brucellosis is characterized by
   A. encephalitis
   B. fluctuating temperature
   C. dysentery
   D rose rash
   E. hepatitis

929. P. pestis is transmitted by
   A. rat flea
   B. dog bite
   C. vaccines
   D. fecal contamination of water
   E. food contamination

930. Undulant fever is caused by microorganisms of the genus
   A. Brucella
   B. Corynebacterium
   C. Shigella
   D. Scarlatina
   E. Hemophilus

931. Negri bodies are minute bodies found in persons or animals infected with
A. tuberculosis
B. diphtheria
C. scarlet fever
D. typhoid fever
E. rabies

932. Tularemia is transmitted by
A. a bite of infected flies and ticks
B. mosquito bites
C. droplet transmission
D. direct contact with convalescent patients
E. bite of rat lice

933. Penicillins are rarely combined with other antibiotics because of
A. potential for toxicity
B. high potential for physical incompatibility
C. high potential for chemical incompatibility
D. danger of potentiation
E. diminished effectiveness

934. Cholera is characterized by
A. dehydration of the tissues
B. bubos
C. erythema of the skin
D. dysentery
E. respiratory paralysis

935. Mumps in children usually involves
A. salivary glands
B. tonsils and throat
C. sex glands
D. pancreas and liver
E. CNS

936. Gray patches on the tonsils or mucous membrane of the nose and throat are associated with
A. measles
B. mumps
C. diphtheria
D. german measles
E. tetanus

937. Concerning the plague
   A. it is transmitted by the rat flea or rat louse
   B. the fleas are natural hosts
   C. organism is never found in the tissues or exudates of those infected
   D. immune serum is administered during infection
   E. Haffkine's vaccine confers absolute immunity

938. Toxoids are
   A. obtained from culture filtrates of viable organisms
   B. bacterial vaccines
   C. nonspecific protein filtrates
   D. nonantigenic toxins
   E. unofficial toxins

939. Koplik's spots are associated with
   A. tularemia
   B. Rocky Mountain spotted fever
   C. diphtheria
   D. measles
   E. scarlet fever

940. Hetacillin is converted by the body to
   A. ampicillin
   B. penicillin G
   C. penicillin V
   D. oxacillin
   E. carbenicillin

941. Which anthelminthic is effective against multiple infestations?
   A. Tolnaftate (Tinactin)
   B. Griseofulvin (Fulvicin)
   C. Tetracycline (Achromycin V)
   D. Flucytosine (Anconbon)
   E. Thiobendazole (Mintezol)

942. Which of the following does NOT apply to S. typhi?
   A. Ferments dextrose, amltose, mannitol, without gas production
   B. Motile
   C. Gram negative
   D. Sensitive to chloromycetin
   E. Ferments lactose and sucrose with gas production

943. A prevalent recent type of bacterial contamination in drugs is from
   A. streptococcus
   B. salmonella
   C. influenza virus
   D. St. Louis encephalitis
   E. rickettsia

944. The proper interpretation of a positive reaction to a tuberculin test is that the person is
   A. suffering from active tuberculosis
   B. immune to invasion by the tubercle bacillus
   C. susceptible to invasion by the tubercle bacillus
   D. sensitive to tuberculo-protein by virtue of previous or present infection
   E. none of the above

945. Athlete's foot is caused by
   A. bacteria
   B. viruses
   C. rickettsia
   D. parasitic worms
   E. fungi

946. Carbenicillin is used primarily to treat infections caused by
   A. P. aeruginosa and proteus
   B. streptococcal infections
   C. resistant staphylococci
   D. meningococci
   E. spirochetes

947. Clindamycin is prone to cause
   A. constipation
   B. severe colitis
   C. sensitivity to light
   D. tooth discoloration
   E. peptic ulcer

948. The Sabin vaccine is superior to Salk vaccine because it
   A. imparts permanent immunity
   B. is genetically unstable
   C. can be administered orally
   D. requires fewer injections
   E. is more readily available

949. Coupled with the stepwise transport of electrons from various oxidizable substances to oxygen, is a most important cellular process called
   A. alcoholic fermentation
   B. formation of coenzymes
   C. oxidative phosphorylation
   D. transamination
   E. hydrogenation

950. Streptococcus viridans is associated with
   A. myositis, cystitis, arthritis
   B. pyorrhea alveolaris, subacute bacterial endocarditis, urinary tract infection
   C. scarlet fever, erysipelas, septic sore throat
   D. meningitis, arthritis, conjunctivitis
   E. furunculosis, carbuncle, lung abscess

951. The only recognized reservoir of meningococcus is
   A. sheep
   B. infected swine
   C. rodents
   D. man
   E. household pets

952. The animal reservoirs of tularemia in the United States are chiefly
   A. rodents and semiaquatic mammals
   B. dogs and other canines
   C. house pets
   D. fowl and game birds
   E. mites and ticks

953. An advantage of cleocin over lincocin is that it
   A. has a much broader spectrum
   B. is bacteriocidal rather than bacteriostatic
   C. is less likely to cause diarrhea
   D. does not produce resistant strains
   E. requires less frequent dosing

954. Rifampin is most useful in treating
   A. gonorrhea
   B. meningococcal infections
   C. fungal infestations
   D. pulmonary tuberculosis
   E. typhoid fever

955. The time of day when fevers tend to peak is
   A. 2 to 4 PM
   B. 4 to 6 AM
   C. 6 to 10 PM
   D. 10 to 12 PM
   E. 10 to 12 AM

956. Ampicillin may give a false-positive diagnostic test for
   A. uric acid
   B. glucose
   C. cholesterol
   D. bilirubin
   E. biliverdin

957. The genus Clostridium are noted for all being
   A. normally harmless GI saprophytes
   B. spore-forming rods dependent to a greater or lesser degree on anaerobiosis
   C. motile by bipolar flagella
   D. possessed of a capsule composed of D-galactose polymer
   E. neurotoxic

958. Epidemic typhus is caused by
   A. rickettsia
   B. viruses
   C. bacteria
   D. molds or yeasts
   E. none of the above

959. Which of the following antibiotics has exceptionally good antifungal action?
   A. Bacitracin
   B. Spectinomycin (Trobicin)
   C. Tobramycin (Nebcin)
   D. Candicidin (Candeptin)
   E. Polymyxin (Aerosporin)

960. A mordant is used as
   A. an agent inducing death
   B. a decolorizing solution for acid-fast organisms
   C. a substance that fixes bacterial stain so the material will retain it
   D. selective stain for capsules
   E. none of the above

961. In order to kill spores
   A. autoclave for 15-20 minutes at 120°C
   B. steam the medium for 15-20 minutes
   C. raise temperature slowly to 90°C and maintain this temperature for 1 hour
   D. heat 15-30 minutes at 100°C in moist heat on 3 successive days
   E. A and B

962. Which of the following is an antibiotic which is very similar to the cephalosporins?
   A. Doxycycline
   B. Minocycline
   C. Amdinocillin
   D. Carbenicillin
   E. Moxalactam

963. The incubation period of rabies in man is
   A. 2-4 weeks
   B. 1-3 weeks
   C. 1-2 months
   D. up to 1 year
   E. up to 2 years

964. The word antibiotic means
   A. bacteriological enzyme
   B. antigrowth substance
   C. bacteriostatic substance produced by micro-organisms
   D. A and B
   E. B and C

965. Clindomycin interacts with
   A. oral anticoagulants
   B. narcotic analgesics
   C. most laxatives
   D. lactose
   E. kaolin

966. Which of the following is NOT an integral part of the growth sequence of a bacterial colony?
   A. Lag phase
   B. Acceleration phase
   C. Exponential phase
   D. Sporulation phase
   E. Death phase

967. A disease NOT produced by a virus is
   A. septic sore throat
   B. smallpox
   C. rabies
   D. mumps
   E. yellow fever

968. Moxan (moxalactum) is most closely related to which of the following classes of antiinfectives?
   A. Aminoglycosides
   B. Tetracyclines
   C. Sulfonamides
   D. Cephalosporins
   E. Oleandomycins

969. Spectinomycin (Trobicin) is used primarily as an alternative to
A. bacitracin
B. penicillin G
C. streptomycin
D. kanamycin
E. cephalosporins

970. Shigella are usually classified by
A. fermentation reactions
B. antigenetic characters
C. combination of A and B
D. phage typing
E. dye tolerance

971. A rickettsial disease which can become an epidemic through infected lice is
A. typhoid
B. poliomyelitis
C. scarlet fever
D. typhus
E. chickenpox

972. A prevalent side effect of Novobiocin is
A. ringing in the ears
B. visual impairment
C. urticaria
D. constipation
E. kidney blockage

973. Most food poisoning is caused by species of
A. typhus
B. salmonella
C. shigella
D. tetanus
E. pasteurella

974. Which of the following are most effective in treating rickettsial infections, generally?
A. Penicillins
B. Tetracyclines
C. Sulfonamides
D. Aminoglycosides
E. Cephalosporins

975. The treatment of choice for leprosy is
A. penicillin therapy
B. broad-spectrum antibiotic therapy
C. chloromycetin therapy
D. sulfone therapy
E. none of the above

976. Which of the following exhibit significant leprostatic activity?
A. Aminoglycosides
B. Cephalosporins
C. Quinacrines
D. Sulfones
E. Pheniramines

977. In the course of an attack of dysentery, the organism is best recovered from
A. the blood stream at peak of fever
B. biopsy of rectal mucosa
C. the stool mucus
D. the urine
E. the saliva

978. Antigen is
A. any foreign material introduced into the human body
B. only protein in nature
C. contained in serum injected in vaccination
D. any protein and few microbiological polysaccharides
E. all of the above

979. Which of the following is NOT a classification of viruses?
A. Dermatropic
B. Neurotropic
C. Viscerotropic
D. Neoplastic
E. Somatophilic

980. An advantage of rabies immune globulin over anti-rabies serum (equine) is
    A. greater effectiveness
    B. lower incidence of adverse reactions
    C. greater immunity to all type of rabies
    D. faster action
    E. longer protection

981. Which of the following is NOT produced by molds?
    A. Penicillin
    B. Terramycin
    C. Streptomycin
    D. Bacitracin
    E. Neomycin

982. Inactivated polio virus vaccine (Salk) should be
    A. pink suspension
    B. white suspension
    C. clear and colorless solution
    D. clear and pink or red solution
    E. clear, straw-colored solution

983. Yellow fever is
    A. transmitted by the body and head louse
    B. found mainly in temperate climates
    C. transmitted by the female Anopheles mosquito
    D. capable of causing a viral disease in epidemic proportions
    E. prevented by means of a vaccine extremely stable to heat and light

984. Agglutinins are
    A. antitoxins which lyse bacteria
    B. carbohydrates
    C. a product of bacterial secretions
    D. antibodies which cause bacteria to clump together
    E. nonspecific

985. By sterilization is meant
    A. freeing an object from life of any kind
    B. removal of organisms capable of causing infection
    C. inhibition of growth of bacteria
    D. removal of facultative anaerobes
    E. none of the above

986. Drug fastness may be attributed to
   A. inferior quality of drug
   B. chemical changes of the drug brought about by the bacteria
   C. mutant forms of the original bacterial strain
   D. use of wrong drug
   E. none of the above

987. Which of the followingis used exclusively for urinary tract infections?
   A. Pyrimethamine (Daraprim)
   B. Metronidazole (Flagyl)
   C. Ticarcillin (Ticar)
   D. Nalidixic acid (Neg Gram)
   E. Cefaclor (Ceclor)

988. Bacterial cells that exhibit acid-fast properties differ from other bacterial cells by
   A. containing nucleoproteins
   B. not differing chemically
   C. high concentration of fatty acids
   D. presence of mycolic acid in combination with waxy material
   E. C and D

989. The action of Clostridium botulinum in disease is due to
   A. number of living bacteria
   B. presence of clostridium in intestines
   C. exotoxin ingested
   D. endotoxins produced
   E. A and B

990. Viruses and rickettsiae differ from bacteria in their food requirements because they
   A. can only live on synthetic media
   B. can only multiply in the presence of bacteria
   C. need sunlight for growth
   D. cannot survive without the presence of living tissue
   E. can only grow in soil

991. Which of the following is usually associated with high incidence of concomitant premenigitis?
    A. Peritonsillar abscess
    B. Otitis media
    C. Quinsy
    D. Cervical adenitis
    E. Pneumonitis

992. Cephapirin has which of the following advantages over cephalothin?
    A. Causes less phlebitis
    B. Gives much higher blood levels
    C. Detoxified more readily
    D. No advantage
    E. A, B, and C

993. Which of the following is very effective in treating amebiasis?
    A. Emetine hydrochloride
    B. Miconazole
    C. Trimethoprim
    D. Vidarabine
    E. Cephaloridine

994. Reactions of antigens with antibodies are
    A. slow
    B. rare
    C. impossible
    D. controlled by temperature
    E. highly specific

995. Thermal death point takes place when
    A. all bacteria of a given species are killed after 10 minutes exposure
    B. all bacteria of a given species are killed after 20 minutes exposure
    C. all bacteria are killed instantaneously
    D. half of the virulent organisms are killed
    E. lysis of bacteria begins

996. Vancomycin should be well diluted to minimize
   A. thrombophlebitis
   B. chance of overdosing
   C. GI problems
   D. agranulocytosis
   E. ear damage

997. Metronidazole is used mainly to treat
   A. resistant staph
   B. syphilis
   C. gonorrhea
   D. trichomonas
   E. pneumonia

998. Rifampin (Rifamycin) is used mainly to treat
   A. resistant staphylococcal infections
   B. septicemia
   C. tuberculosis
   D. pneumonia
   E. venereal diseases

999. Trench mouth is caused by
   A. B. vincentii
   B. Leptospira
   C. S. aureus
   D. E. coli
   E. none of the above

1000. Paralytic polio
   A. is more common in temperate than tropical zones
   B. can be readily cured
   C. is no longer seen
   D. is more common now than 5 years ago
   E. is caused by a bacteria

1001. Autogenous vaccines are
   A. vaccines prepared from autotropic bacteria
   B. prepared from autolytic organisms
   C. prepared from patient's own organisms
   D. identical with stock vaccines
   E. administered for passive immunization

1002. Bacterial antigens
- A. are vectors of disease
- B. are antibiotic substances
- C. may be demonstrated in the specific antibacterial serum
- D are used to produce active immunity
- E. never produce disease

1003. Which of the following has the longest serum half-life?
- A. Doxycycline
- B. Demeclocycline
- C. Tetracycline
- D. Oxytetracycline
- E. Methacycline

1004. Chloroquine (Araien) is given at which of the following intervals as a prophylactic for malaria?
- A. Monthly
- B. Weekly
- C. Biweekly
- D. Daily
- E. Four hour

1005. Active immunization against diphtheria may be developed by injections with
- A. alum-precipitated culture
- B. antitoxin
- C. filtrates of C. Hoffmanni and C. Xerosis cultures
- D. toxoid
- E. antidiphtheritic serum

1006. In young children, tetracyclines often cause
- A. agranulocytosis
- B. discoloration of teeth
- C. conjunctivitis
- D. muscular weakness
- E. hyperplasia of the gums

1007. The etiology agent of mononucleosis is
   A. Epstein-Barr virus
   B. betahemolytic streptococcus
   C. resistant staphylococcus
   D. a rickettsia
   E. a fungus

1008. Which of the following drugs should NOT be used to treat malaria in patients who have a history of psoriasis?
   A. Chloraquine
   B. Primaquine
   C. Quinine
   D. Quinacrine
   E. Pyrimethamine

1009. An advantage of iodophors over iodine solutions is
   A. increased antiseptic activity
   B. easier application
   C. they do not stain
   D. less pain on wounds
   E. none of the above

1010. Passive immunity is the result of
   A. injection with the specific antigen
   B. injection with the specific antibody
   C. a lack of response to the antigen
   D. partial immunization
   E. recovery from a specific infection

1011. Immunization against measles usually employs
   A. a measles toxoid
   B. gamma globulin
   C. a live virus
   D. live bacteria
   E. attenuated rickettsia

1012. Influenza vaccines seldom produces hypersensitivity because they are
   A. not prepared in eggs
   B. mixed with preservatives
   C. hypoallergenic extracts
   D. given in such low doses
   E. highly purified

1013. Alpha hemolysis
   A. causes dissolution of phagocytes
   B. cannot be demonstrated in the absence of complement
   C. is characteristic of D. pneumoniae
   D. is characteristic of scarlet fever strains of streptococci
   E. is best demonstrated on chocolate agar plates

1014. Interferon is
   A. an enzyme
   B. a protein complex
   C. an agglutinogen
   D. a precursor of amino acids
   E. none of the above

1015. The incubation period for mumps in humans is usually
   A. 14-21 days
   B. 7-14 days
   C. 1-7 days
   D. 15-28 days
   E. 21-30 days

1016. Which of the following is used specifically to treat gonorrhea?
   A. Novobiocin
   B. Spectinomycin
   C. Viomycin
   D. Cycloserine
   E. Cephazolin

1017. Nitrofurantoin (Furadantin) is used mainly to treat
   A. upper respiratory tract infections
   B. urinary tract infections
   C. pneumococcal infection
   D. syphilis
   E. rickettsial infections

Match the following:

A. Infectious jaundice
B. Typhus
C. Malaria
D. Syphilis
E. Chanacroid

1018. Treponema pallidum
1019. Leptospira ictero hemorrhagica
1020. Rickettsia prowazeki
1021. Hemophilus ducreyi
1022. Plasmodium vivax

Match each of the numbered drugs with the lettered drug interaction:

A. Dissulfiram
B. Cefotoxamine
C. Cholestryramine
D. Gentamycin
E. Oral neomycin

1023. Penicillin G
1024. Carbenicillin
1025. Penicillin V
1026. Bacampicillin
1027. Aziocillin

1028. Pathogenic staphylococci in carriers are usually harbored in
A. nose and skin
B. gastrointestinal tract
C. kidney and bladder
D. salivary glands
E. all of the above

1029. An organ of the body that is often damaged permanently by rheumatic fever is the
A. lung
B. kidney
C. heart
D. liver
E. spleen

1030. A variety of Staphylococcus aureus that is very resistant to heat is
A. caloris
B. communis
C. theramophilus
D. lactophilus
E. globigii

1031. The route of administration of bacitracin is
A. IV
B. IM
C. topical
D. oral
E. all of the above

1032. Gas gangrene is commonly caused by
A. Pasteurella
C. Clostridia
C. Rickettsia
D. Shigella
E. Mycobacteria

1033. Which of the following is any pus-forming skin infection?
A. Dermatitis
B. Empyema
C. Emphysema
D. Pyoderma
E. Coryza

1034. The organism(s) causing urinary tract infections is(are)
A. E. coli
B. Proteus vulgaris
C. Pseudomonas aeruginosa
D. Staphylococcus pyogenes
E. all of the above

1035. The mechanism of dry heat sterilization is primarily
A. oxidation
B. reduction
C. coagulation
D. denaturation
E. none of the above

1036. Bacillary dysentery is usually caused by which of the following organisms?
A. Pasteurella
B. E. coli
C. Shigella
D. Plasmodium
E. Ascaria

1037. Untreated gonorrhea in the female may cause
A. discoloration of teeth
B. abortion
C. increased incidence of carcinoma
D. sterility
E. fungal infections

1038. The preferred method of sterilization for mineral oil is
A. autoclaving
B. bacterial filtration
C. gas sterilization
D. dry heat
E. radiation

1039. Which of the following should be used for severe, potentially fatal fungal infections?
A. Nystatin
B. Griseofulvin
C. Amphotericin B
D. Candidicin
E. Gentian violet

1040. Thrush is caused by a(an)
A. rickettsia
B. streptococcus
C. staphylococcus
D. fungus
E. virus

1041. All of the following "toxins" are typical of all pathogenic staphylococci EXCEPT
A. hemolysin
B. leukocidin
C. enterotoxin
D. coagulase
E. emolosin

1042. Bacteriophages are usually
   A. bacteria
   B. viruses
   C. lipoidal
   D. polysaccharides
   E. none of the above

1043. Weil-Felix reaction is a test for
   A. typhus fever
   B. malaria
   C. yellow fever
   D. presence of Clostridium botulinum
   E. none of the above

1044. Histoplasmosis is best treated with
   A. penicillin G
   B. amphotericin B
   C. ampicillin
   D. tetracycline
   E garamycin

1045. An antibody is chemically
   A. a protein
   B. a polysaccharide
   C. an amino acid
   D. any foreign substance in the body
   E. none of the above

1046. Acyclovir (Zovirax) is classified as a(an)
   A. antiviral
   B. antirickettsial
   C. anthelmintic
   D. cephalosporin
   E. penicillin

1047. Scabies is a disease of the
   A. mouth
   B. skin
   C. liver
   D. lungs
   E. GI tract

1048. The most effective drugs against Proteus species are
- A. penicillins
- B. sulfonamides
- C. tetracyclines
- D. nitrofurantoins
- E. erythromycins

1049. Rocky Mountain spotted fever is caused by
- A. a virus
- B. a rickettsia
- C. a bacteria
- D. an amoeba
- E. none of the above

1050. Ethylene oxide sterilizes by a mechanism primarily involving
- A. coagulation
- B. oxidation
- C. alkylation
- D. hydrolysis
- E. denaturation

1051. A pathogenic fungus is
- A. Trichoderma viride
- B. Rhizopus nigricans
- C. Geotrichum candium
- D. Blastomyces dermatitidis
- E. C and D

1052. Gentamicin is commonly used in combination with which of the following to treat serious Pseudomonas infections?
- A. Ampicillin
- B. Penicillin G
- C. Oxacillin
- D. Cephalosporins
- E. Carbenicillin

1053. An antibiotic of therapeutic value is produced by
- A. Penicillium roqueforti
- B. Penicillium chrysogenum
- C. Streptomyces scabies
- D. Aspergillum glaucus
- E. Penicillium italicum

1054. Which of the following organisms is capable of devitalizing living tissue in gas gangrene?

A. C. welchii
B. C. novyi
C. C. septicum
D. C. sporogenes
E. C. histolyticum

1055. Gentamicin closely resembles
A. novobiocin
B. kanamycin
C. penicillin G
D. lincomycin
E. polymyxin B

1056. Bacitracin can be obtained from a strain of
A. E. coli
B. P. aeruginosa
C. B. subtilis
D. S. aureus
E. none of the above

1057. The function of antibodies in immunity is
A. to neutralize toxins
B. entirely bacteriostatic
C. to produce more leukocytes
D. to build up resistance against any infections
E. A and D

1058. Dapsone (DDS) is used primarily to treat
A. Rocky Mountain spotted fever
B. pneumonia
C. leprosy
D. urinary tract infections
E. herpes simplex

1059. Which is best to treat ringworm of the body?
A. Boric acid
B. Tolnaftate
C. Penicillin V
D. Gentamycin
E. Iodoform

1060. A test used to check leakage of bacterial filters is
A. the Seitz test
B. the millipore test
C. the seep test
D. bubble point
E. none of the above

1061. Vancomycin is effective primarily against
A. gram-positive bacilli
B. gram-negative bacilli
C. gram-positive cocci
D. gram-negative cocci
E. encapsulated forms

1062. Rheumatic fever is usually precipitated by
A. virus infections
B. staph infections
C. mycotic infestations
D. streptococcal infections
E. none of the above

1063 The most common location of the organisms in a typhoid carrier is
A. nasopharynx
B. gallbladder
C. epididymis or fallopian tube
D. kidney
E. large bowel and nodes of gut

1064. Which of the following is used commonly to prevent sepsis in severe burn cases?
A. Mafenide (Sulfamylon)
B. Sulfadiazine sodium
C. Sulfisoxazole (Gantrisin)
D. Sulfameter (Sulla)
E. Sulfamethoxazole (Gantanol)

1065. Passive immunity usually gives which of the following protection to the patient?
A. None
B. Complete
C. Long term
D. Short term
E. Undetermined

1066. HEPA filters are widely used in
A. autoclaves
B. laminar flow hoods
C. face masks
D. oxygen masks
E. gas sterilizers

1067. Cephalosporins are
A. vaccines
B. diagnostic test agents
C. antibiotics
D. serums
E. antigens

1068. Hookworm is caused by
A. Ancylostoma duodenale
B. Plasmodium vivax
C. Salmonella typhosa
D. Endamoeba histolytica
E. Trichinella spiralis

1069. Aplitest is used to test for
A. diabetes
B. pregnancy
C. measles
D. tuberculosis
E. whooping cough

1070. A bacteriostatic agent has which of the following effects on bacteria?
A. It kills bacteria on contact
B. It enhances their growth
C. It induces spore formation
D. It inhibits multiplication of bacteria
E. It dehydrates the bacteria

1071. An anaphylactic reaction is an indication of
A. no antibodies present in blood
B. immunity
C. hypersensitivity to given protein
D. presence of typhoid bacilli
E. infestation by Trypanosomes

1072. Nystatin (Mycostatin) is used mainly to treat
   A. blastomycosis
   B. coccidiomycosis
   C. histoplasmosis
   D. candida infections
   E. athlete's foot

1073. Penicillins can be obtained commercially from
   A. yeasts
   B. molds
   C. animal sources
   D. fungi
   E. bacteria

1074. The anthelmintic niclosamide (Niclocide) is most effective against
   A. tapeworms
   B. pinworms
   C. whipworms
   D. hookworms
   E. threadworms

1075. The most important single step in treating gas gangrene is
   A. specific antitoxin
   B. adequate surgical removal of devitalized tissue
   C. systemic antibodies
   D. fever therapy
   E. local antibiotic therapy

1076. The mode of spread of botulinum toxin in the body is by
   A. direct extension along nerve trunks
   B. blood stream spread
   C. lymphatic spread
   D. direct contiguity in the gut wall
   E. all of the above

1077. Vancomycin (Vancocin) is used mainly to treat
   A. urinary tract infections
   B. gonorrhea
   C. skin infections
   D. serious infections resistant to other drugs
   E. burns

1078. Epidemic parotitis is more commonly called
A. flu
B. St. Louis encephalitis
C. common cold
D. mumps
E. measles

1079. Botulism toxin
A. is frequently found in meats
B. comes from an organism found commonly in soil
C. grows well in an acid medium
D. all of the above
E. none of the above

1080. Species of Proteus are implicated in
A. wound infections
B. urinary tract infections
C. peritonitis
D. gastroenteritis
E. all of the above

1081. The disease varicella is commonly known as
A. smallpox
B. measles
C. mononucleosis
D. scarlet fever
E. chickenpox

1082. A fomite is a(an)
A. airborne carrier of disease
B. inanimate object which transmits disease
C. symptom of throat infections
D. means of preventing disease
E. type of immunity

1083. Although normally a harmless saprophyte, E. coli is the most common source of
A. peritonitis
B. cholecystitis
C. acute genitourinary infections
D. pancreatitis
E. appendicitis

1084. An advantage of amoxicillin over ampicillin is that it
A. is more rapidly absorbed
B. is less toxic
C. has a broader spectrum
D. is detoxified more completely
E. has a longer duration of action

1085. A drug used in treating second or third degree burns is
A. mafenide (Sulfamylon)
B. sulfisoxizole (Gantrisin)
C. nitrofurantoin (Furadantin)
D. tetracycline (Achromycin)
E. polymyxin (Aerosporin)

1086. Biavax II is used for immunization against
A. rubella and mumps
B. rubella and measles
C. mumps and measles
D. measles and whooping cough
E. mumps and whooping cough

1087. Which of the following is NOT a characteristic of typhoid fever?
A. Insidious onset, with malaise, anorexia, headache
B. High polymorph leukocytosis and shift to the left
C. Pulse slow compared to fever
D. Rose spots
E. Splenomegaly

1088. A broad spectrum antibiotic that has proven effective against resistant staph infections is
A. Vibramycin
B. minocycline
C. oxytetracycline
D. demeclocycline
E. tetracycline

1089. Urticaria is usually caused by
A. noninfectious bacteria
B. allergy
C. virus
D. rickettsia
E. molds

1090. To produce active artificial immunity, the patient's body
A. is injected with sterile bacterial proteins
B. is injected with sterile bacterial antigens
C. is injected with living infectious organisms with attenuated virulence
D. is induced to produce antibodies against a specific disease
E. all of the above

1091. Suby's Solution G is used for irrigation of the
A. mouth for Vincent's disease
B. lower urinary tract
C. eye
D. ear
E. skin in burn treatment

1092. The poliomyelitis virus ordinarily enters the body through the
A. ear
B. skin
C. mouth
D. lungs
E. none of the above

1093. An example of immunization with attenuated living infectious agent is
A. vaccination
B. anaphylaxis
C. any antigen injection
D. Neisser-Wechsberg phenomenon
E. anabolism

1094. In the United States most cases of botulism can be traced to
A. undercooked pork
B. home-canned sausage and other meats
C. home-canned vegetables and fruits
D. fish from polluted water
E. infected pastry

1095. The organism most commonly found in infections of the bone is
A. Meningococcus
B. E. coli
C. Staphylococcus pyogenes
D. Mycobacterium tuberculosis
E. Pseudomonas aeruginosa

1096. Vaccine prepared from a patient's own infection is called
A. autogenous vaccine
B. stock vaccine
C. monovalent vaccine
D. polyvalent vaccine
E. simple vaccine

1097. The substance in airplant glue most responsible for adverse effects is
A. phenol
B. organic solvent
C. gums
D. alcohol
E. volatile oils

1098. Water is unfit for human consumption when coliform organisms are present because
A. it contains bacteria
B. it shows fecal contamination
C. it indicates possible contamination by entering pathogens
D. B and C
E. none of the above

1099. Which of the following antibiotics is usually given only once daily for maintenance?
A. Declomycin
B. Vibramycin
C. Achromycin
D. Aureomycin
E. Chloromycetin

1100. Which one of the following antifungals also has amebicidal properties?
A. Nystatin (Mycostatin)
B. Flucytosine (Ancobon)
C. Miconazole (Monostat)
D. Metronidazole (Flagyl)
E. Griseofulvin

4. CHEMISTRY

DIRECTIONS: For each of the following multiple choice and matching questions, choose the one most appropriate answer.

1101. Which of the following contains an ethylenediamine nucleus?
   A. Chlortetracycline
   B. Tripelennamine
   C. Lidocaine
   D. Pentobarbital
   E. Pyrvinium pamoate

1102. Aldehydes tend to produce which of the following upon oxidation?
   A. Ketones
   B. Alkanes
   C. Esters
   D. Acids
   E. None of the above

1103. Which of the following is used to test for reducing sugars in urine?
   A. Acetest
   B. Benzidine reagent
   C. Benedict's reagent
   D. Iodine
   E. None of the above

1104. Duquenois reagent, when acidified, produces a blue color in the presence of
A. amphetamines
B. barbiturates
C. LSD
D. marijuana
E. STP

1105. EDTA is
A. a monobasic acid
B. a polybasic acid
C. an imide
D. an ester
E. none of the above

1106. Marquis reagent in the presence of opium alkaloids gives which of the following colors?
A. Red
B. Orange
C. Purple
D. Green
E. Yellow

1107. Strychnine produces which of the following colors in the presence of sulfuric acid and potassium dichromate?
A. Reddish-orange
B. Black
C. Yellow green
D. Blue-violet
E. Brown

1108. A common agent in smoking deterrents is
A. nicotine
B. emetine
C. coal tar
D. phenol
E. lobeline

1109. Trichloromethane is also called
A. methyl chloride
B. carbon tetrachloride
C. chloroform
D. Freon
E. chlorox

1110. Chloral hydrate is usually classified as a(an)
A. acid
B. amhydride
C. ketone
D. aldehyde
E. ester

1111. Which of the following instruments is used to measure sodium and potassium ions quantitatively?
A. Ion chamber
B. Flame photometer
C. Polarimeter
D. Spectrophotometer
E. Friabilator

1112. The principal hydrolysis degradation product of aspirin is
A. salicylic acid
B. methyl salicylate
C. salicylamide
D. acrolein
E. acetyl chloride

1113. Grignard reagents usually contain
A. Co
B. Cu
C. Fe
D. Pb
E. Mg

1114. NMR is used mainly for
A. assays
B. irradiation
C. identification of chemical substances
D. radioisotopes
E. none of the above

1115. Chemically, tetracyclines are
A. acids
B. bases
C. amphoteric
D. nonsalt formers
E. all esters

1116. Stool softeners frequently contain
- A. anionic surfactants
- B. auaternary ammonium compounds
- C. organic acids
- D. sulfonthaleins
- E. aldehydes

1117. When aspirin is heated with water for several minutes, cooled, and a drop or two of ferric chloride TS is added, the color that develops is
- A. blue
- B. red
- C. violet
- D. green
- E. none of the above

1118. pH is usually measured with a
- A. platinum electrode
- B. mercury electrode
- C. copper electrode
- D. glass electrode
- E. none of the above

1119. The principle of the refractometric method of analysis depends upon
- A. densities between two substances
- B. molecular weights of substances assayed
- C. volumes of substances assayed
- D. ultraviolet spectrum of substance being assayed
- E. none of the above

1120. Mercury compounds exert their toxic effects by tying up
- A. sulfhydryl groups
- B. ester linkages
- C. lactones
- D. carboxyl groups
- E. double bonds

1121. The visible range of light has a wave-length range of
- A. 1000-6000 angstroms
- B. 4000-7000 angstroms
- C. 40-70 millimicrons
- D. 10-60 millicrons
- E. 700-1100 angstroms

1122. How many molecules of NaOH will react with 6.06×10^{23} molecules of sulfuric acid?
   A. 6.06×10^{23}
   B. 12.12×10^{23}
   C. 3.03×10^{23}
   D. 6.06×10^{46}
   E. $6.06 \times 10^{11.5}$

1123. An 18-carbon atom saturated fatty acid is
   A. myristic acid
   B. lauric acid
   C. oleic acid
   D. stearic acid
   E. none of the above

1124. Sucrose hydrolyzes to
   A. glucose
   B. glucose and mannose
   C. glucose and galactose
   D. glucose and fructose
   E. glucose and lactose

1125. Which of the following contains 16 carbon atoms?
   A. Arachidic acid
   B. Oleic acid
   C. Stearic acid
   D. Aspirin
   E. None of the above

Match the following ions with the characteristic color given in the flame test:

   A. Green
   B. Blue
   C. Brick red
   D. Violet
   E. Yellow

1126. Calcium
1127. Barium
1128. Lead
1129. Potassium
1130. Sodium

Match the following chemical names with the correct common name:

A. Ether USP
B. Glycerin
C. Toluene
D. Chloroform
E. Phenol

1131. Hydroxybenzene
1132. Trichloromethane
1133. Diethyl oxide
1134. Symmetrical trihydroxy propane
1135. Methyl benzene

1136. Which of the following salts would be acid in reaction when dissolved?
A. Sodium lactate
B. Magnesium carbonate
C. Antimony chloride
D. Sodium chloride
E. Potassium sulfate

1137. The ionization constant of water at 25°C is
A. 7
B. 14
C. 1×10^{-7}
D. 1×10^{7}
E. 1×10^{-14}

1138. Barbiturates containing a sulfur atom are usually
A. ultra short-acting
B. unpredictable
C. short-acting
D. intermediate-acting
E. long-acting

Match the following ions with their respective specific tests:

A. Flame test
B. Diphenylthiocarbazone
C. 8-hydroxyquinoline
D. Vapor-litmus paper test
E. None of the above

1139. Zinc
1140. Barium
1141. Strontium
1142. Calcium
1143. Ammonium

Match the following:

A. Equal volumes of gases under the same conditions of temperature and pressure contain the same number of molecules
B. The volume of a gas is inversely proportional to pressure if the temperature is constant
C. The pressure exerted by a gas is proportional to the absolute temperature if the volume of gas is kept constant

1144. Boyle's law
1145. Avogadro's law
1146. Charles' law

1147. Le Chatelier's law of mobile equilibrium states that "if the conditions of a system in equilibrium are altered, . . .
A. equilibrium cannot be reestablished"
B. the equilibrium shifts in the direction which tends to neutralize the change in conditions"
C. the equilibrium shifts in the direction which tends to accentuate the change in conditions"
D. there is no change in the equilibrium"
E. none of the above

Match each substance with its pH in aqueous solution:

A. Acid
B. Alkaline
C. Neutral

1148. Sodium carbonate
1149. Phenol
1150. Potassium chloride
1151. Sodium pentobarbital

Match each substance with its primary classification:

A. Barbiturate
B. Aldehyde
C. Ester
D. Nonionic surfactant

1152. Aspirin
1153. Thioamytal
1154. Polysorbate 80
1155. Chloral hydrate

Match the following:

A. Conjugate base of HCl
B. Ionic or molecular substance capable of giving up a proton to another substance
C. Conjugate base of NH_{4+}
D. 1 g molecular weight of reagent dissolved in 1000 g of solvent
E. Proton acceptor

1156. Acid
1157. Base
1158. Cl^-
1159. NH_3
1160. Molal solution

Match each group or type of drugs with the cation or anion with which it is most closely associated:

A. Mg
B. Organic nitrates
C. Cobalt
D. Potassium
E. Gold
F. Iron

1161. Hematinics
1162. Antiarthritics
1163. Treatment of muscle weakness
1164. Treatment of angina
1165. Antineoplastics
1166. Antacids

1167. Chromium is an important trace element needed for
A. blood formation
B. vitamin absorption
C. glucose metabolism
D. fat metabolism
E. protein metabolism

Match each of the following substances with its chemical classification:

A. Ketone
B. Polyhydric alcohol
C. Fluorinated hydrocarbon

1168. Freon II
1169. Glycerin
1170. Acetone

Match the following:

A. Ratio of absolute viscosity in poises to the density
B. Based upon reflection of light
C. Force of friction that tends to retard movement in a fluid body
D. Based upon absorption of light

1171. Viscosity
1172. Nephelometry
1173. Colorimetry
1174. Kinematic viscosity

1175. Adsorption is a(an)
A. irreversible chemical reaction
B. reversible chemical reaction
C. complexation phenomenon
D. light-induced reaction
E. physical phenomenon

Match each organic acid with the appropriate therapeutic use:

A. Antiseptic
B. Burn treatment
C. Irrigation
D. Fungistatic
E. Acne treatment
F. Sunscreen
G. Vitamin

1176. Acetic acid
1177. Ascorbic acid
1178. Boric acid
1179. Tannic acid
1180. Undecylenic acid
1181. Transretinoic acid
1182. Paraaminobenzoic acid

1183. London forces in molecules are
A. coordinate covalent bonds
B. weak intramolecular forces
C. strong intermolecular forces
D. weak intermolecular forces
E. hydrogen bonds

Match the following:

A. d, 1-amphetamine
B. 2 or more compounds with same molecular formula but differing in at least one chemical or physical property
C. Used to calculate molecular weights
D. Colorless form of a dye
E. Change in optical rotation of a solution of an optically active compound
F. Increased attraction between molecules as the number of atoms increases
G. 2 isomers that rotate plane polarized light equal amounts in the opposite direction

1184. Leuco base
1185. Freezing point
1186. Isomers
1187. Racemic mixture
1188. Mutarotation
1189. Van der Waals force
1190. Enantiomorphs

1191. Fluorinated hydrocarbons are often used as
A. general anesthetics
B. hypnotics
C. antiarrhythmics
D. antihypertensives
E. diuretics

1192. Protein hydrolysates consist mainly of
A. enzymes
B. enzyme acids
C. nitrites
D. amino acids
E. nitrates

1193. A reagent used to test for indole structures is
A. dimethyl ketone
B. formic acid
C. p-aminobenzaldehyde
D. acetaldehyde
E. benzoic acid

1194. The rate of zero order reactions
- A. changes constantly
- B. is independent of temperature
- C. is independent of concentration
- D. holds only for light-catalyzed reactions
- E. holds only for radioactive compounds

1195. A normal solution contains
- A. 1 g equivalent weight of solute in 1000 g of solution
- B. 1 g equivalent weight of solute in 1000 cc of solvent
- C. 1 g equivalent weight of solute in 1000 cc of solution
- D. 1 g molecular weight of solute in 1000 cc of solvent
- E. 1 g molecular weight of solute in 1000 cc of solution

1196. Determination of iodine value depends upon
- A. substitution with iodine for the hydrogen in the fatty acids
- B. addition of iodine at the double bond of fatty acids
- C. oxidation of the fatty acids by iodine
- D. analysis of the iodine content of a fatty acid
- E. none of the above

1197. Most of the local anesthetics are
- A. esters of salicylic acid
- B. esters of p-aminobenzoic acid
- C. amides of naphthoic acid
- D. esters of propionic acid
- E. allantoin derivatives

1198. The pH of solutions of sodium borate tends to be
- A. strongly acidic
- B. weakly acidic
- C. neutral
- D. weakly alkaline
- E. strongly alkaline

1199. Deuterium is a radioactive form of
- A. carbon
- B. oxygen
- C. hydrogen
- D. iodine
- E. cobalt

1200. A saccharimeter measures
- A. light transmittance
- B. optical rotation
- C. light absorption
- D. refractive index
- E. none of the above

1201. Ester types of local anesthetics are primarily metabolized by
- A. cholinesterase
- B. oxidation
- C. reduction
- D. amylases
- E. liver esterases

1202. A common active ingredient of some cough preparations is
- A. glyceryl guaicolate
- B. sorbitol
- C. sodium metabisulfite
- D. thimerosal
- E. amaranth

1203. Clathrates are
- A. cage-like complexes
- B. chelates
- C. sandwich-type complexes
- D. Pi bond complexes
- E. ligands

1204. The most successful sulfonamides have what type of substitution on the amido nitrogen?
A. Carboxylic
B. Alicyclic
C. Electropositive
D. Electronegative
E. Aliphatic

1205. Cholestyramine (Questran) causes a number of drug interactions because it is
A. very acid in pH
B. a complexing agent
C. a solubilizer
D. very alkaline in pH
E. carrier substance

Match the following:

A. Cleocin
B. Klebcil
C. Garamycin

1206. Gentamicin
1207. Clindamycin
1208. Kanamycin

A. RCOONa
B. RCOCl
C. $RCOOC_2H_5$
D. $RCONH_2$
E. $(RCO)_2O$

1209. Salt
1210. Ester
1211. Acid anhydride
1212. Acyl halide
1213. Acyl amide

Match the correct ingredient with the following pharmaceutical preparations:

A. Hydrochloric acid
B. Chlortrimeton
C. Boric acid
D. Iodine
E. Pectin
F. Zinc undecylenate
G. Zirconium salt
H. Glyceryl guaiacolate
I. Albamycin
J. Cetamium

1214. Lugol's solution
1215. Desenex
1216. Acidulin
1217. Ziradryl
1218. Robitussin
1219. Collyrium
1220. Coricidin
1221. Kaopectate
1222. Formula 44 cough syrup
1223. Panalba

1224. In preparations used for gastric distress alumium hydroxide combines antacid action with
A. laxative action
B. coating action
C. diuretic action
D. histamine antagonist action
E. preservative action

1225. The principal oxidation product of ethylene glycol is
A. ethanol
B. citric acid
C. carbon monoxide
D. oxalic acid
E. acetaldehyde

5. BIOCHEMISTRY

DIRECTIONS: For each of the following multiple choice and matching questions, choose the one most appropriate answer.

1226. A diagnostic agent used primarily for visualization of the lympathic system is
   A. isosulfan blue
   B. radioactive iodine
   C. barium sulfate
   D. diododrast
   E. methyl red

1227. Which is NOT an essential amino acid?
   A. Threonine
   B. Tryptophane
   C. Valine
   D. Glutamine
   E. Methionine

1228. Insulin is usually classified as a(an)
   A. protein
   B. amino acid
   C. phospholipid
   D. enzyme
   E. hormone

1229. An enzyme is a substance which
A. hydrolyzes
B. dehydrates
C. converts heat to energy
D. acts as a catalyst
E. is changed chemically in a reaction

1230. A substance found commonly in fermented foods which can be toxic when MAO inhibitors are used is
A. ADP
B. STP
C. tyramine
D. histidine
E. phenylalanine

1231. Man is most sensitive to which of the following tastes?
A. Sour
B. Sweet
C. Bitter
D. Salty
E. Alkaline

1232. Which of the following is needed in determining the isoelectric point of an amino acid?
A. Structural formula
B. Dissociation constant
C. Electrophoretic pattern
D. Composition
E. pH

1233. The conversion of an amino acid to a sugar is
A. hydrolysis
B. cocarboxylation
C. glycolysis
D. glucogenesis
E. none of the above

1234. MAO is classified as a(an)
A. protein inhibitor
B. complexing agent
C. enzyme
D. hormone
E. amino acid

1235. With which of the following tests does the anticonvulsant carbamazepine interfere?
A. Glucose tolerance test
B. Pregnancy test
C. Thyroid function test
D. Blood uric acid test
E. White blood cell count

1236 Which substance yields the largest number of calories per gram?
A. Carbohydrates
B. Proteins
C. Minerals
D. Fats
E. Vitamins

1237. The lethal effect of CO is due to its
A. vapor pressure
B. H_2O solubility
C. ability to form CO_2 easily
D. ability to combine with hemoglobin
E. ability for forming a stable complex with myoglobin

1238. Which ions are involved in uptake of renal stones?
A. Iron and cobalt
B. Sodium and potassium
C. Calcium and sodium
D. Chloride and bicarbonate
E. Chloride and oxalate

1239. The principal site of glucose production in the human body is the
A. blood
B. pituitary gland
C. muscle tissue
D. liver
E. small intestine

1240. Which of the following drugs is LEAST likely to cause electrolyte imbalance?
A. Chlorothiazide
B. Aluminum hydroxide
C. Potassium chloride
D. Ethacrynic acid
E. Sodium bicarbonate

1241. The coenzymes of the dehydrogenases include all of the following EXCEPT
A. DPN
B. coenzyme II
C. FAD
D. apoenzyme
E. FMN (flavin adenine mononucleotide)

1242. Deficiency of folic acid will cause
A. anemia
B. rickets
C. night blindness
D. beriberi
E. diabetes

1243. A component of coenzyme A is
A. inosine
B. thiamine
C. pantetheine
D. triphosphopyridine nucleotide
E. acetate

1244. Epinephrine and norepinephrine are synthesized from
A. glycine
B. argenine
C. phenol
D. catechol
E. tyrosine

1245. The major buffer of the extracellular fluid is
A. bicarbonate-CO_2 system
B. phosphate
C. protein
D. sodium
E. none of the above

1246. An excess of nitrogenous waste in the blood causes
A. acidosis
B. alkalosis
C. kidney stones
D. uremia
E. none of the above

1247. The normal blood chemistry value of sodium in serum in mg% is
A. 310-340
B. 50-100
C. 18-20
D. 390-450
E. 25-40

1248. Which may give a false + in the 5-HIAA tests for carcinoma?
A. NaCl
B. Glyceryl guaiacolate
C. KCl
D. Tetracycline
E. Ampicillin

1249. The active proteolytic enzyme in gastric juice is
A. pepsinogen
B. pepsin
C. bilirubin
D. trypsin
E. secretin

1250. A negative nitrogen balance could occur
A. during normal pregnancy
B. in malnutrition
C. during normal child growth
D. during convalescence
E. none of the above

1251. Which of the following enhances activity of azathioprine by inhibiting enzymatic oxidation?
A. Allopurinol
B. Elase
C. Dipyridamole
D. Trimethoprim
E. Tranylcypromine

1252. Which of the following is NOT an enzyme involved in glycolysis?
A. Enolase
B. Diaphorase
C. Glycerophosphate dehydrogenase
D. Pyruvate kinase
E. Hexokinase

1253. The end-product of the hydrolysis of glycogen is
A. galactose
B. mannose
C. glucose
D. xylose
E. arabinose

1254. Porphyrins are involved in the building of
A. bones
B. teeth
C. muscle
D. blood
E. scar tissue

1255. Sincalide (Kinevac) is used as a diagnostic aid to obtain samples of
A. albumen
B. gastric juice
C. blood sugar
D. bile
E. ketones

1256. A normal value for glucose in blood is
A. 250-350 mg%
B. 200-250 mg%
C. 100-200 mg%
D. 80-120 mg%
E. 50-75 mg%

1257. Which of the following will displace coumarin from binding sites?
A. Insulin
B. Norepinephrine
C. Acetylcholine
D. Tolbutamide
E. Ephedrine

1258. Between the particulate and micellar constituents of cells there exists an aqueous phase which contains
A. soluble proteins
B. organic substances such as glucose
C. cellular active products such as creatine
D. electrolytes
E. all of the above

1259. Which may give a false + glucose with Tes-Tape?
A. Vitamin B_1
B. Vitamin E
C. Tetracycline
D. Erythromycin
E. Vitamin C

1260. Which of the following is classified as a polysaccharide?
A. Saccharin
B. Starch
C. Lactose
D. Sodium cyclamine
E. Maltose

1261. In the typical cell, the mitochondria contains
A. cytochrome oxidase
B. succinic acid oxidase
C. cytochrome C
D. all of the above
E. none of the above

1262. The main carbohydrate of the blood is
A. d-fructose
B. mannitol
C. d-glucose
D. sorbitose
E. 1-glucose

1263. The presence of mitochrondria in living cells can be determined by the use of
A. neutral red
B. methylene blue
C. janus green
D. phenolpthalein
E. none of the above

1264. The diagnostic agent Hemachek is used to test for
   A. occult blood
   B. white blood cell count
   C. red blood cell count
   D. monocyte count
   E. blood hemoglobin

1265. Which drug is likely to elevate the value in the PBI test?
   A. Lithium carbonate
   B. INH
   C. Disulfiram
   D. Aspirin
   E. Potassium iodide

1266. The only disaccharide synthesized in human metabolism is
   A. maltose
   B. lactose
   C. fructose
   D. cellulose
   E. erythrose

1267. A deficiency of which of the following vitamins can cause night blindness?
   A. D
   B. K
   C. A
   D. E
   E. B complex

1268. Progesterone is derived mainly from
   A. estrone
   B. testosterone
   C. corpus luteum
   D. chorionic gonadotropin
   E. thyroxine

1269. The conversion of beta-carotene to vitamin A is carried out in the
   A. liver
   B. pancreas
   C. spleen
   D. thymus
   E. adrenal cortex

1270. The heat-labile factor in the vitamin B complex is
A. riboflavin
B. biotin
C. thiamine
D. folic acid
E. niacin

1271. Blood clotting can be prevented by
A. sodium chloride
B. potassium chloride
C. sodium citrate
D. lithium chloride
E. all of the above

1272. Which is most likely to elevate the value of a BUN test?
A. Tetracycline
B. Penicillin G
C. Benzathine penicillin
D. Ampicillin
E. Cromolyn sodium

1273. Pancreatin is used therapeutically for
A. coughs
B. pneumonia
C. cystic fibrosis
D. kidney failure
E. cirrhosis

1274. Which of the following is present in all connective tissue?
A. Mucoids
B. Lipids
C. Albuminoid
D. All of the above
E. None of the above

1275. Phytonadione (vitamin K_1) is used to treat
A. hematuria
B. cystic fibrosis
C. hemorrhagic disease of newborn
D. agranulocytosis
E. leukemias

1276. In the electrophoretic process at a pH below the isoelectric point, a protein will
A. migrate to negative pole
B. migrate to positive pole
C. exhibit no migration
D. form a Zwitter ion
E. none of the above

1277. Colchicine can give false-positive tests for
A. glucose
B. uric acid
C. urates
D. ketones
E RBC

1278. Keratin is a(an)
A. protein
B. albuminoid
C. glutelin
D. peptone
E. histone

1279. The pellagra-preventive factor in the vitamin B complex is
A. inositol
B. pantothenic acid
C. riboflavin
D. niacin
E. paraaminobenzoic acid

1280. Vitamin K is necessary for
A. prevention of rickets
B. prevention of pernicious anemia
C. formation of prothrombin
D. formation of DNA
E. muscle tone

1281. Which of the following furnishes much energy to muscles?
A. ACTH
B. LSD
C. RNA
D. DNA
E. ATP

1282. Oral contraceptives exert their effect primarily by
A. preventing fertilization of the egg
B. suppressing ovulation
C. inactivating sperm
D. preventing menses
E. none of the above

1283. Fatty acid oxidation in humans is mediated by
A. ozone
B. amylases
C. tryptophan
D. glucuronidase
E. coenzyme A

1284. A combination of L-Dopa and which of the following will cause depletion of catecholamines?
A. Carbidopa
B. Amantadine
C. Chlorpromazine
D. Riboflavin
E. A and B

1285. The Benzidine test is used to test for
A. uric acid
B. alkaloids
C. amino acids
D. blood
E. lipids

1286. Betazole is used for clinical testing of
A. thyroid function
B. gastric secretion
C. glucose tolerance
D. liver function
E. kidney function

1287. The follicle-stimulating hormone (prolactin) and the interstitial cell-stimulating hormone are produced by
A. islets of Langerhans
B. thymus gland
C. thyroid gland
D. pineal gland
E. pituitary gland

1288. Which of the following is capable of either releasing dopamine or delaying its destruction?
A. Trihexyphenidyl
B. Benztropine
C. L-Dopa
D. Orphenadrine
E. Amantadine

1289. Removal of which glands results in low calcium level in blood and leads to tetany and death?
A. Thyroid
B. Endocrine
C. Adrenal
D. Parathyroid
E. None of the above

1290. The average life of a red blood cell is about
A. 7 days
B. 14 days
C. 3 weeks
D. 1-2 months
E. 4 months

1291. The precursors of vitamin A are
A. proteins
B. tocopherols
C. ergosterols
D. carotenes
E. calciferols

1292. Defects in purine metabolism can cause
A. gout
B. rheumatoid arthritis
C. anemia
D. methhemoglobinemia
E. malnutrition

1293. The usual source of heparin is
A. blood
B. fish
C. tissues of domestic mammals
D. plants
E. synthetic

1294. The protein precursor of thyroxine is
A. ornithine
B. threonine
C. tryptophan
D. thyroglobulin
E. thyroxinogen

1295. Methyldopa interferes with analysis for
A. occult blood in urine
B. glucose in urine
C. ketones in urine
D. urinary catecholamines
E. uric acid

1296. Iron in the form of ferritin is stored in the
A. liver
B. intestinal mucosa
C. spleen
D. bone marrow
E. all of the above

1297. Gigantism and acromegaly are diseases attributed to malfunction of
A. pineal gland
B. thymus gland
C. islets of Langerhans
D. pituitary gland
E. gonads

1298. Sensi-slide is used to test for
A. renal impairment
B. hyperglycemia
C. hypoglycemia
D. pregnancy
E. ulcers

1299. Most nitrogen heterocycles are detoxified by
A. methylation
B. reduction
C. oxidation
D. hippuric acid
E. transconversion

1300. The feeding of vitamin B_{12} to pernicious anemia patients overcomes
- A. the lack of intrinsic factor
- B. the lack of extrinsic factor
- C. lack of hydrochloric acid production
- D. folic acid deficiency
- E. all of the above

1301. Approximately what percentage of the population are Rh positive?
- A. 30%
- B. 50%
- C. 60%
- D. 85%
- E. 95%

1302. The fat soluble vitamins are
- A. B complex, C, and D
- B. A, D, E, and K
- C. A, B, C, and D
- D. B complex, E, and K
- E. A, B complex, and D

1303. Fick's law deals with
- A. passive diffusion
- B. viscosity
- C. transamination
- D. active transport
- E. protein synthesis

1304. To avoid pituitary hypofunction which of the following therapies should be discontinued gradually?
- A. Diphenylhydantoin
- B. Potassium chloride
- C. ACTH
- D. Primidone
- E. Trimethadione

1305. The enzyme carbonic anhydrase is markedly inhibited by
- A. salicylates
- B. phenolic compounds
- C. sulfonamides
- D. fluorides
- E. malonates

1306. Zymogens are inactive forms of
A. proteins
B. lipids
C. vitamins
D. genes
E. enzymes

1307. The human body stores vitamin A in
A. the liver
B. the spleen
C. the intestine
D. fat depots
E. muscle tissue

1308. The metabolic degradation of hemoglobin takes place principally in
A. the reticuloendothelial system
B. the RBC
C. the liver cells
D. the kidney tubules
E. all of the above

1309. The metabolic breakdown of hemoglobin in the mammal involves
A. the formation of bile pigments
B. no oxidative cleavage of the porphyrin ring
C. the formation of urobilinogen
D. the formation of biliverdin
E. all of the above

1310. The nonprotein portion of hemoglobin consists of
A. 3 heme units surrounding a n iron atom
B. 4 heme units surrounding a ferric atom
C. a ferrous complex of protoporphyrin IX
D. 4 pyrrole rings linked through a ferric molecule
E. none of the above

1311. The amino acid that is an important precursor of hemoglobin is
A. alanine
B. proline
C. glycine
D. leucine
E. histidine

1312. In most mammals, except man and the higher apes, uric acid is metabolized by
   A. reduction to ammonia
   B. oxidation to allantoin
   C. degradation to nitrogen
   D. hydrolysis to ammonia
   E. oxidation to ammonia and carbon dioxide

1313. Muscarine mimics the action of
   A. serotonin
   B. hyaluronidase
   C. acetylcholine
   D. cysteine
   E. norepinephrine

1314. In man, the major nitrogenous excretion product is
   A. amino acids
   B. ammonia
   C. nitrogen
   D. purines and pyrimidines
   E. none of the above

1315. Protirelin is used to test for
   A. kidney stones
   B. brain damage
   C. gastric secretion
   D. catecholamines in urine
   E. thyroid function

1316. Which vitamin is used occasionally as an antioxidant?
   A. Vitamin D
   B. Vitamin K
   C. Vitamin B_1
   D. Vitamin E
   E. Vitamin B_3

1317. Which of the following is responsible for the transfer of genetic information?
   A. ATP
   B. RNA
   C. DNA
   D. STP
   E. None of the above

1318. Tromethamine (Tham) is used to treat
   A. thyroid deficiency
   B. acidosis
   C. alkalosis
   D. acromegaly
   E. schizophrenia

1319. Ptyalin is a(an)
   A. lipase
   B. anhydrase
   C. urease
   D. amylase
   E. proteinase

1320. The mineral zinc is most important for
   A. blood cell formation
   B. bone formation
   C. oxidative processes
   D. normal growth
   E. muscle contractions

1321. An important enzymatic reaction involved in muscular contraction is
   A. glucose-6-phosphatase reaction
   B. glycogenolysis
   C. ATP-creatine transphosphorylase reaction
   D. enolase reaction
   E. all of the above

1322. Death due to cyanide poisoning results from
   A. cyanide-hemoglobin complex formation
   B. cyanide combining with the red blood cell
   C. cyanide inhibiting cytochrome oxidase
   D. coronary vessel occlusion
   E. none of the above

1323. Total parenteral nutrition (TPN) include amino acids, carbohydrates, fats, electrolytes, minerals, and
   A. animal protein
   B. vitamins
   C. dehydrocholic acid
   D. choline esterase
   E. none of the above

1324. The physiological importance of hemoglobin lies in its ability
A. to combine irreversibly with oxygen and carbon dioxide
B. to combine reversibly with oxygen at the ferric portion of the molecule
C. to combine irreversibly with oxygen at the ferrous portion of the molecule
D. to combine reversibly with oxygen at the ferrous portion of the molecule
E. none of the above

1325. Elevation of blood uric acid levels tends to produce
A. dizziness
B. dyspnea
C. hypertension
D. muscular weakness
E. gout

1326. High doses of vitamin C may interfere with testing for which of the following in the urine?
A. Creatinine
B. Glucose
C. Uric acid
D. Chloride
E. Albumen

1327. The visual impulse is associated with the
A. photochemical transformation of rhodopsin
B. the reduction of TPN
C. the condensation of opsin with vitamin C
D. the hydrolysis of visual purple
E. all of the above

1328. The biochemical role of the carotenoids lies in their conversion to
A. folic acid
B. folinic acid
C. ascorbic acid
D. vitamin A
E. none of the above

1329. Which of the following stimulates hepatic microsomal enzymes?
A. Phenacemide
B. Mannitol
C. Phenobarbital
D. Urea
E. ASA

1330. Which of the following vitamins has a structure similar to the steroids?
A. C
B. B_1
C. A
D. D
E. K

1331. A synthetic form of vitamin K is
A. calciferol
B. tocopherol
C. biotin
D. menadione
E. cholesterol

1332. Drugs containing hydroxyl or carboxyl groups are detoxified by
A. hippuric acid
B. glucuronic acid
C. acetylation
D. reduction
E. hydrolysis

1333. Collagenase is an enzyme used to
A. repair muscle
B. debride skin in burn cases
C. increase digestion
D. enhance absorption
E. hydrolize fats

1334. Passive diffusion requires what kind of energy?
A. None
B. High
C. Low
D. Kinetic
E. Electrical

1335 Which of the following drugs are absorbed mainly from the stomach?
A. Alkaline
B. Neutral
C. Acidic
D. All of the above
E. None of the above

1336. The nucleic acids, RNA and DNA, play important roles in the biosyntesis of protein. A sugar inherent in their structure is
A. glucose
B. sucrose
C. fructose
D. sorbose
E. none of the above

1337. Glycogenesis takes place mainly in the
A. pancreas
B. blood
C intestine
D. spleen
E. liver

1338. It has been shown that an important step in the metabolism of epinephrine and norepinephrine is
A. oxidation of the amino group by cytochrome oxidase
B. reduction of the side chain
C. hydrolysis of the amino group
D. o-methylation
E. oxidation of the catechol nucleus

1339. Although the prostaglandins are hormone-like, they more closely resemble which of the following chemically?
A. Proteins
B. Carbohydrates
C. Enzymes
D. Lipids
E. Porphyrins

1340. Which of the following neurons transmit impulses from sensory to motor neurons?
A. Afferent
B. Glial
C. Microglial
D. Internuncial
E. Efferent

1341. Some tissues form lactic acid under aerobic conditions. This phenomenon, especially characteristic of tumor tissues, is termed
A. aerobic glycolysis
B. lactation
C. oxidation
D. oxidative-phosphorylation
E. none of the above

1342. The pyridine nucleotides, DPN and TPN, are essential cofactors in the metabolism of many substances. An important part of the structure of these molecules is
A. vitamin A
B. vitamin C
C. nicotinamide
D. vitamin E
E. all of the above

1343. Magnesium deficiencies are usually associated with
A. growth retardation
B. mental disease
C. parkinsonism
D. impaired muscular contraction
E. acromegaly

1344. The incidence of side effects from L-Dopa approaches
A. 25%
B. 50%
C. 75%
D. 100%
E. none of the above

1345. Aerobic oxidation of carbohydrates is mediated via
A. the urea cycle
B. the tricarboxylic acid cycle
C. the pentose-phosphate shunt
D. Embden-Myerhof pathway
E. all of the above

1346. Which of the following would have little effect on rate absorption of a drug?
A. Strength
B. pH
C. Active transport
D. Particle size
E. Crystalline form

1347. Phenytoin causes elevated blood glucose levels by
A. enhancing degradation of insulin
B. increasing glucose absorption
C. increasing glucagon release
D. decreasing insulin release
E. B and C

1348. Most normal values in urinalysis are based on
A. mg or g per 100 ml
B. g/l
C. mg%
D. g/24-h excretion
E. none of the above

1349. Taste perception requires which of the following trace metals?
A. Chromium
B. Iron
C. Manganese
D. Zinc
E. Cobalt

1350. Prostaglandins are closely related to
A. hormones
B. fat-soluble vitamins
C. dibenzazepines
D. tocopherols
E. amino acids

6. PHYSIOLOGY AND PATHOLOGY

DIRECTIONS: For each of the following multiple choice and matching questions, choose the one most appropriate answer.

1351. A patient in a diabetic coma
   A. may have the odor of acetone on his breath
   B. may be perspiring profusely
   C. usually recovers without treatment
   D. may twitch excessively
   E. none of the above

1352. One of the most potent stimulants of the respiratory center is
   A. increased pO_2 in the blood
   B. decreased pO_2 in the blood
   C. an increased pCO_2 in the blood
   D. decreased pCO_2 in the blood
   E. none of the above

1353. A substance present in the small intestine which inhibits gastric secretion is
   A. enterokinin
   B. histamine
   C. enterogastrone
   D. enterokinase
   E. none of the above

1354. One of the physiological effects of an increased CO_2 in the blood is
   A. increased dissociation of oxyhemoglobin
   B. increased mental activity
   C. decreased respiration
   D. decreased dissociation of oxyhemoglobin
   E. none of the above

1355. Metabolic acidosis may be brought about by
   A. loss of CO_2 by increased ventilation
   B. retention of CO_2 brought about by respiratory obstruction
   C. persistent vomiting
   D. absorption of excessive amount of $NaHCO_3$
   E. none of the above

1356. The P wave of the electrocardiogram is associated with
   A auricular repolarization
   B. auricular contraction
   C. auricular depolarization
   D. ventricular repolarization
   E. none of the above

1357. The A wave of the venous pulse is caused by
   A. auricular contraction which impedes blood flow in the large veins
   B. incoming blood which stagnates during ventricular systole
   C. the thrust of blood into the aorta which is transmitted to the large veins
   D. an abnormally constricted vena cava
   E. none of the above

1358. The disintegration of the platelets gives rise to a factor required for normal blood coagulation. This factor is
   A. thromboplastin
   B. thrombin
   C. prothrombin
   D. fibrinogen
   E. none of the above

1359. A condition in which there is a decrease in urine excretion is called
A. anuria
B. polyuria
C. oliguria
D. uropenia
E. cytosuria

1360. Osgood-Schlatter's syndrome is commonly seen in
A. infants
B. elderly people
C. Asian races
D. preschoolers
E. early teens

1361. Contraction of the heart is initiated by the
A. SA node
B. AV node
C. bundles of His
D. left atrium
E. right ventricle

1262. Drugs which stimulated the parasympathetic branch of the autonomic nervous system are called
A. anticholinergics
B. adrenergic agents
C. cholinergic agents
D. cholinolytic agents
E. sympathomimetics

1263. The most frequent cause of angina pectoris is
A. coronary atherosclerosis
B. coronary insufficiency
C. cardiac fibrillation
D. cardiac congestion
E. lack of conduction

1264. The respiratory center is located in the
A. cerebrum
B. cerebellum
C. hydothalamus
D. medulla
E. pons

1365. A major factor in control of sodium excretion by the kidney is
A. aldosterone
B. testosterone
C. ptyalin
D. circulation
E. coenzyme A

1366. When a series of repetitive stimuli are applied with a rate high enough to cause summation of contraction, the muscle is said to be in a state of
A. rigor
B. tetanus
C. irreversible contracture
D. fatigue
E. none of the above

1367. In young adults, normal blood pressure is
A. 100/60
B. 80/80
C. 140/90
D. 120/120
E. 120/80

1368. Histotoxic hypoxia usually results from
A. monoxide poisoning
B. high altitude
C. anemia
D. decreased utilization of oxygen
E. bends

1369. Systemic diastolic pressure depends largely upon
A. cardiac output
B. elasticity
C. peripheral resistance
D. A and B
E. B and C

1370. The glomerulus is
A. a network of capillaries
B. a lymph node
C. a large artery entering the kidney
D. a dilator substance produced by the kidney
E. none of the above

1371. Henle's loop is found in the
 A. liver
 B. stomach
 C. intestine
 D. kidney
 E. inner ear

1372. A lack of speech coordination is
 A. dysphasia
 B. paresthesia
 C. dyspnea
 D. diplopia
 E. dyspraxia

1373. The effect of adrenocortical hormone on the kidney
 A. icnreases the rate of sodium resorption and potassium excretion
 B. decreases the rates of sodium resorption and potassium excretion
 C. increases the rate of sodium and potassium resorption
 D. decrease the rate of sodium and potassium resorption
 E. none of the above

1374. The macrophages of CNS tissue are
 A. microglia
 B. neurilemma
 C. arachnoid villi
 D. folia
 E. microsoma

1375. The fundamental unit or organized neural activity is the
 A. ganglion
 B. reflex arc
 C. synpase
 D. afferent neuron
 E. efferent neuron

1376. A substance used to measure the glomerular filtration rate is
- A. insulin
- B. inulin
- C. diodrast
- D. paraaminohippuric acid
- E. none of the above

1377. The antidiuretic hormone is secreted from
- A. kidney cortex
- B. kidney medulla
- C. anterior pituitary
- D. posterior pituitary
- E. none of the above

1378. The effect of the antidiuretic hormone is to
- A. decrease water loss by the lungs
- B. increase perspiration
- C. decrease the rate of resorption of water by the kidney
- D. increase the rate of resorption of water by the kidney
- E. none of the above

1379. The sympathetic ganglia are located
- A. near the heart
- B. near the spinal cord
- C. near the adrenal glands
- D. near the tissues they innervate
- E. in the extremities

1380. The cardiac reserve is
- A. the maximal percentage increase in cardiac output that can occur
- B. the amount of blood remaining in the heart after systole
- C. the volume of blood the heart can hold
- D. the volume of blood within the walls of the cardiac musculature that can be called upon in an emergency
- E. none of the above

1381. A substance generally used for measuring renal plasma flow is
A. ethyl alcohol
B. inulin
C. paraaminohippuric acid
D. glucose
E. none of the above

1382. The endocrine glands differ from ordinary glands because
A. they are larger
B. they are smaller
C. they secrete substances
D. they all have the same shape
E. they are ductless

1383. The chemical mediator released at the end of the parasympathetic nerve fiber is
A. acetylcholine esterase
B. acetylcholine
C. epinephrine
D. norepinephrine
E. amino oxidase

1384. An endocrine gland that plays an important role in calcium metabolism is
A. pancreas
B. hypophysis
C. thyroid
D. parathyroid
E. gonads

1385. Heat cramps are due primarily to loss of
A. water
B. body temperature
C. lithium
D. potassium
E. sodium

1386. The quantity of hemoglobin in 100 ml of blood averages:
A. 5 g
B. 10 g
C. 15 g
D. 20 g
E. none of the above

1387. The term hematocrit means the percentage of the
A. blood that is red blood cells
B. blood that is plasma
C. blood volume to the extracellular space
D. new blood formed every 120 days
E. none of the above

1388. The most important functional process that the neutrophils and monocytes carry out is
A. phagocytosis
B. IDK
C. tachyphylaxis
D. urea absorption
E. none of the above

1389. The uppermost portion of the intestine is the
A. cecum
B. jejunum
C. ileum
D. duodenum
E. colon

1390. The pigment which gives the urine its color is
A. urochrome
B. bilirubin
C. biliverdin
D. urobilin
E. none of the above

Match the following substances with the organ or gland secreting each:

A. Anterior pituitary
B. Adrenals
C. Pancreas
D. Stomach mucosa
E. Thyroid

1391. Epinephrine
1392. Lactogenic hormone
1393. Insulin
1394. Thyroxine
1395. Gastrin
1396. Testosterone
1397. ACTH

1398. Cor pulmonale is
A. obstruction of the lung
B. decrease in RBC
C. hypertrophy of the right ventricle
D. decrease in WBC
E. increase in WBC

1399. Equalization of air pressure between the tympanic cavity and the outside atmosphere is done by the
A. stapes
B. cochlea
C. eustachian tube
D. anvil
E. semicircular canal

1400. Which of the following inhibits gastric acid secretion?
A. Vagal stimuli
B. Neurotensin
C. Gastrin
D. Protein meals
E. Calcium ion

1401. Which of the following substances of the spinal cord serves as a conducting pathway for impulses?
A. Gray matter
B. White matter
C. Cerebrospinal fluid
D. Pia mater
E. Arachnoid

1402. Fibrinogen is synthesized mainly in the
A. blood
B. pancreas
C. kidney
D. liver
E. lung

1403. A prevalent long-term danger in extensive burn cases is
A. infections
B. gangrene
C. convulsions
D. hypothermia
E. hyperthermia

1404. The neurotransmitter released at the end of the sympathetic nerve fiber is
A. epinephrine
B. norepinephrine
C. acetylcholine
D. acetylcholine esterase
E. amine oxidase

1405. Drugs which cause dilation of the eye pupil are
A. miotics
B. mydriatics
C. cycloplegics
D. antispasmodics
E. anorectics

1406. The most common blood type is
  A. A
  B. B
  C. O
  D. AB
  E. X

1407. Addison's disease is caused by dysfunction of
  A. posterior pituitary
  B. adrenal medulla
  C. adrenal cortex
  D. parathyroids
  E. bone marrow

1408. Fever during infection is due to
  A. increased heat production, followed by decreased heat loss
  B. decreased heat loss, followed by increased heat production
  C. an action of bacterial pyrogens independent of the body's heat-control mechanisms
  D. a functional hyperthyroidism due to irritation of the thyroid and release of colloid
  E. none of the above

1409. Moderate stretch of cardiac muscle
  A. strengthens the contractile force
  B. weakens the contractile force
  C. has no effect on the contractile force
  D. abolishes contraction
  E. initiates contraction

1410. The O_2 dissociation curve of hemoglobin is shifted to the right by
  A. decreased CO_2
  B. increased CO_2
  C. increased pH
  D. increased N_2 tension
  E. decreased N_2 tension

Match each of the following with a function each performs in the body:

A. Oxygen transport
B. Defense against infection
C. Regulation of pressure
D. Nutrition of fetus
E. Regulates heart rate
F. Balance
G. Electrical transmitter
H. Night vision

1411. Labyrinth
1412. Rods
1413. Umbilical cord
1414. Hemoglobin
1415. WBC
1416. Carotid sinus
1417. Vagus
1418. AV node

1419. The bundles of His are found in the
A. lung
B. intestines
C. liver
D. heart
E. kidney

1420. The pacemaker of the heart is the
A. coronary artery
B. right ventricle
C. SA node
D. AV node
E. left ventricle

1421. The chief danger of any drug causing respiratory stimulation is
A. liver damage
B. the chance of inducing convulsions
C. kidney damage
D. induction of hypotension
E. induction of hypertension

1422. Which of the following substances is the source of energy in nerve fibers?
A. Potassium
B. Sodium ion
C. Calcium ion
D. Glucose
E. Magnesium ion

1423. Rales are
A. lesions
B. visual disturbances
C flashing pains
D. abnormal chest sounds
E. none of the above

1424. Hodgkin's disease is usually centered in the
A. central nervous system
B. GI system
C. musculoskeletal sustem
D. lymphatic system
E. blood

1425. Which of the following substances is filtered but not reabsorbed by the tubules?
A. Xylose
B. Plasma proteins
C. Inulin
D. NaCl
E. Paraaminohippurate

1426. The Chick-Martin test is used to test for efficiency of
A. coumarins
B. heparin
C. antibiotics
D. blood clotting
E. analgesics

1427. The principal action of lymph glands is
A. to destroy microorganisms
B. as a warning system
C. to reduce fever
D. to filter out solids
E. none of the above

1428. Diverticulosis is usually associated with the
- A. stomach
- B. small intestine
- C. liver
- D. skin
- E. colon

1429. The sensory ganglion of the brain stem is the
- A. cerebral cortex
- B. hypothalamus
- C. thalamus
- D. medulla
- E. basal ganglia

1430. Large doses of radiation (600-800R) are very likely to cause
- A. nausea and vomiting
- B. sterility
- C. bone marrow depression
- D. all of the above
- E. none of the above

1431. When light rays come to a focus behind the retina, the eye is said to be
- A. hypermetropic
- B. presbyopic
- C. astigmatic
- D. myopic
- E. emmetropic

1432. Progressive fibrosis and scarring of the liver are known as
- A. diverticulitis
- B. diverticulosis
- C. hepatitis
- D. cirrhosis
- E. ulcerative colitis

1433. Major constituents of bile are
- A. nonelectrolytes
- B. organic acids
- C. organic bases
- D. micelles
- E. inorganic bases

1434. Histoplasmosis is caused by an internal invasion of the body by
A. viruses
B. fungi
C. helminths
D. bacteria
E. rickettsia

1435. The first heart sound is the result of
A. the closure of the semilunar valves
B. closure of the auriculoventricular valves
C. the rapid inflow of blood from auricle into ventricle
D. inflow of blood from ventricle into the aorta
E. none of the above

1436. Parietal cells secrete
A. sodium bicarbonate
B. hydrochloric acid
C. insulin
D. bile salts
E. ACTH

1437. The respiratory stimulant effect of CO_2 is due to a direct action on the
A. carotid body
B. carotid sinus
C. aortic body
D. respiratory center
E. none of the above

1438. The ion in highest concentration in the cells is
A. Na
B. Mg
C. K
D. Ca
E. Fe

1439. The ion in highest concentration outside the cells is
A. Na
B. Mg
C. K
D. Ca
E. Fe

1440. Heavy metals exert their toxic effects in the body by
A. blocking enzymes
B. sclerosing tissues
C. precipitating proteins
D. depressing oxygen exchange
E. none of the above

1441. A term denoting dryness of the mouth is
A. zerophthalmia
B. stomatitis
C. xerostomia
D. xerotocia
E. xeromenia

1442. Polycythemia is characterized by
A. anemia
B. high WBC
C. high RBC
D. low RBC
E. eosinophilia

1443. The most important cardiac and vasomotor centers are situated in the
A. hypothalamus
B. medulla
C. cerebrum
D. cerebellum
E. none of the above

1444. Most of the venous CO_2 is in the form of
A. carbonate
B. carbonic acid
C. bicarbonate
D. dissolved CO_2
E. none of the above

1445. A sudden increase in arterial blood pressure causes
A. an increase in heart rate
B. a fall in venous pressure
C. reflex bradycardia
D. reflex hyperpnea
E. reflex increase in venous pressure

1446. A hormone released by the presence of fat in the duodenum and which causes contraction of gall-bladder muscle is
A. secretin
B. pancreolipase
C. cholecystokinin
D. corticotropin
E. gonadotropin

1447. The pH of the blood is the pH of
A. the cells
B. the plasma
C. the average of cell and plasma
D. the difference between cell and plasma
E. none of the above

1448. Bilirubin is produced by
A. biosynthesis
B. the kidney
C. hemoglobin decomposition
D. decomposition of bile salts
E. the spleen

1449. Which of the following transport(s) urine to the bladder?
A. Urethra
B. Ureters
C. Glomeruli
D. Loop of Henle
E. None of the above

1450. The main function of the gallbladder is to
A. secrete bile
B. concentrate bile
C. eliminate bile
D. biosynthesize bile
E. none of the above

1451. Dextrans are sometimes used clinically to treat
- A. diabetes mellitus
- B. diabetes insipidus
- C. severe shock
- D. leukemias
- E. anemias

1452. Trench foot should never be treated by
- A. elevation
- B. immersion in warm water
- C. penicillin
- D. cool air
- E. wrapping

1453. If all other factors remain constant, the velocity of blood flow in the aorta is
- A. greater than the pulse wave velocity
- B. approximately equal to the pulse wave velocity
- C. inversely proportional to aortic diameter
- D. directly proportional to the square of the aortic diameter
- E. independent of the left ventricular minute volume

1454. Vincent's angina is a disease of the
- A. heart
- B. coronary artery
- C. veins
- D. mouth
- E. none of the above

1455. Dysphagia is defined as
- A. earache from any cause
- B. painful menstruation
- C. toothache
- D. difficulty swallowing
- E. painful eye inflammation

Match each of the following with its characteristic effect:

A. Raises, increases or elevates
B. Lowers, depresses or decreases
C. Has no effect

1456. Epinephrine on blood pressure
1457. Morphine on size of the eye pupil
1458. Edecrin on potassium levels
1459. Dehydration on urine output
1460. Atropine on salivary secretions
1461. Bile salts on absorption
1462. Infections on WBC
1463. MAO inhibitors on serotonin levels
1464. Morphine on bowel movements
1465. Iron on WBC

1466. The sinoatrial node is stimulated by
A. the myogenic reflex
B. the preganglionic sympathetic endings
C the postganglionic sympathetic endings
D. the preganglionic parasympathetic endings
E. none of the above

1467. Repeated transfusions of whole blood can frequently produce
A. megaloblastic anemias
B. pernicious anemias
C. iron overload
D. allergic reactions
E. bone marrow depression

1468. Crohn's disease is a disease of the
A. brain
B. spinal cord
C. stomach
D. colon
E. kidney

1469. Discs are associated with the
A. brain
B. feet
C. spinal column
D. arms
E. taste buds

1470. The most prevalent type of white blood cells are the
A. lymphocytes
B. eosinophils
C. basophils
D. neutrophils
E. monocytes

1471. Tetany in hypoparathyroidism is caused by
A. high pH of serum
B. high calcium
C. low phosphorus
D. low calcium
E. high phosphorus

1472. Methyl testosterone is a hormone of the
A. corpus luteum
B. follicle
C. interstitial cells
D. pituitary
E. placenta

1473. Nystagmus is a condition associated with the
A. eyes
B. ears
C. colon
D. kidney
E. liver

1474. Secretion of adrenal cortical hormones is primarily controlled by
A. somatotropic hormone
B. epinephrine
C. glucagon
D. ACTH
E. ICSH

1475. Most patients suffer from acute renal failure as a result of
A. dehydration
B. nitrosis
C. cirrhosis
D. bacterial infection
E. hyperkalemia

1476. The adrenal steroid corticosterone action is primarily concerned with
   A. water balance
   B. salt metabolism
   C. carbohydrate metabolism
   D. basal metabolism
   E. calcium metabolism

1477. Gamma globulin is
   A. a protein fraction of the blood
   B. the portion of the blood that may be removed by centrifuging
   C. the part of the blood removed by the clot
   D. the part of the blood that is soluble in trichloracetic acid
   E. the part of the blood that cannot be salted out with ammonium sulfate

1478. The part of the eye that is concerned with eye focus is (are) the
   A. cones
   B. rods
   C. iris
   D. lens
   E. eye muscle

1479. The lung is covered by the
   A. bronchioles
   B. alveolar sac
   C. pleura
   D. alveoli
   E. cartilage

1480. The sympathetic system receives its connection with the central nervous system from which area?
   A. Cranial nerves
   B. Thoracic spinal cord
   C. Thoracolumbar spinal cord
   D. Lumbar spinal cord
   E. Lumbopelvic spinal cord

1481. Which of the following percentages represents the extracellular portion of total body water?
A. Approximately 33%
B. Approximately 20%
C. Approximately 50%
D. Approximately 75%
E. Approximately 10%

1482. An inflammation of the kidney substance and pelvis is
A. pyelonephritis
B. hepatitis
C. pyemesis
D. pyometritis
E. perichondritis

1483. The electrocardiogram reveals the time of conduction from the sinoatrial node to the subendocardial ventricular muscle by the length of
A. QRS interval
B. QT interval
C. PR or PQ interval
D PT interval
E. RS interval

1484. The villi are found in the
A. small intestine
B. large intestine
C. stomach
D. esophagus
E. none of the above

1485. Acid rebound is associated with the use of
A. total parenteral nutrition
B. undecylenates
C. histamine antagonists
D. purgatives
E. antacids

1486. A wasting due to lack of nutrition to a body part is
A. atrophy
B. hypertrophy
C. aplasia
D. hyperplasia
E. gerontopia

1487. A sphygmomanometer is used to measure
- A. lung capacity
- B. blood pressure
- C. basic metabolic rate
- D. electrical impulses of the heart
- E. temperature

1488. The human cell has how many chromosomes?
- A. 24
- B. 46
- C. 48
- D. 96
- E. none of the above

1489. Which of the following conditions may be based on genetic predisposition?
- A. Exfoliative dermatitis
- B. Dermatitis medicamentosa
- C Lichen planus
- D. Psoriasis
- E. Atopic dermatitis

Match each of the following substances with the function it measures in terms of renal clearance:

- A. Tubular
- B. Glomerular
- C. Tubular and glomerular

1490. PAH
1491. PAH + inulin
1492. Inulin

1493. The breast bone is called the
- A. sternum
- B. thorax
- C. ribs
- D. ulna
- E. femur

1494. Dyspnea means
   A. painful muscle spasm
   B. pain in the heart
   C. pain in extremities
   D. painful breathing
   E. none of the above

1495. Cystitis is an inflammation of the
   A. ovary
   B. vagina
   C. urethra
   D. kidney
   E. bladder

1496. Blood makes up about which fraction of body weight?
   A. 1/5
   B. 1/10
   C. 1/15
   D. 1/20
   E. 1/30

1497. Sickle cell anemia is characterized by
   A. lack of iron
   B. lack of B_{12}
   C. abnormal shape of red blood cells
   D. lack of folic acid
   E. megaloblastic red blood cells

1498. Another term for hypsophobia is
   A. acrophobia
   B. dipsophobia
   C. polyphobia
   D. hydrophobia
   E. dysphobia

1499. The longest muscle in the body is the
   A. abductor longus
   B. gluteus maximus
   C. transversus abdominus
   D. psoas major
   E. sartorius

1500. Insulin and which of the following are secreted in the islets of the pancreas?

A. Trypsin
B. Glucose
C. Glucagon
D. Luteinizing hormone
E. None of the above

EXPLANATORY ANSWERS

The author has made every effort to thoroughly verify the answers to the questions which appear on the preceding pages. However, as in any text, some inaccuracies and ambiguities may occur; therefore, if in doubt, please consult your references.

The Publisher

1. (A) This is a mixture of electrolytes.

2. (C) Tweens favor o/w emulsions because of high HLB.

3. (B) The energy required for a molecule of drug to leave the lattice is considerably less for the amorphous form.

4. (C) Roller mills are most useful with semisolids.

5. (B) Particle size reduction is used mainly to increase wetability.

6. (A) All other types exhibit decreased viscosity under stress.

7. (A) 4.55 gr = 1%
   3.0 gr = X% than X = 0.66%

8. (D) It is a form of vitamin B_{12}.

9. (C) Spans merely contain fewer oxyethylene groups than tweens.

10. (B) Filtering will not break emulsions, but the other methods will.

11. (B) Not always true, but not uncommon.

12. (A) Oral doeses are metabolized by the liver before reaching systemic circulation.

13. (B) This is the usual evidence of decomposition (oxidation).

14. (B) 473/5000 x 1000 = 95 mg

15. (C) It potentiates the antidiuretic activity of vasopressin.

16. (E) Stability and solubility properties may be changed.

17. (E) Drug will be changed or eliminated before diffusion is attained.

18. (C) This is a measure of degree of pressurization.

19. (C) This is a measure of exposure to radioactivity.

20. (C) It is a mercaptopurine derivative.

21. (B) Phenol is miscible with water below the 10% level or above 90%.

22. (B) It is the negative log of the hydrogen ion concentration (or hydronium ion conc).

23. (E) Muscle tissue is the only one of the three that seldom stores drugs.

24. (B) When a drug is stored, this value increases rapidly.

25. (B) It initiates or improves uterine contractions.

26. (B) Hydrolysis of penicillin G is rapid.

27. (E) All three properties are affected and all contribute to enhanced absorption.

28. (A) This diuretic fluoresces significantly.

29. (D) Protein binding ties up the drug and makes it un available for biotransformation.

30. (B) The combination of sodium phosphate and acetate salts combines both prompt onset and sustained action.

31. (C) Many enteric coatings do not reliably release the drug.

32. (C) This is a synonym.

33. (C) Sulfonylurea antidiabetics increase metabolism of digitoxin.
34. (A) Phenytoin reduces plasma levels of methadone
35. (B) Additive CNS depression occurs.
36. (E) Intensity of blockade and duration of action is increased.
37. (D) Urea increases excretion of lithium, thus decreasing blood levels.

38. (D) Diminishes chalky taste.

39. (C) Other media do not promote growth as well.

40. (C) If not diluted, a false negative result is common.

41. (D) Thioglycollate is a good medium to show growth.

42. (D) They produce hepatic enzyme induction.

43. (E) The reason is to increase solubility.

44. (E) The nitrate ion must be converted to nitrite ion.

45. (E) 6/6+12 (390 mg) = 130 mg

46. (A) This drug gives up water of hydration easily.

47. (C) Vinblastine and vincristine are the drugs obtained from this plant.

48. (A) This method would provide about twice as much drug as is needed.

49. (A) The drug must be highly un-ionized to penetrate the blood brain barrier and this process is quite slow in general.

50. (D) Used to prevent degradation before the site is reached.

51. (E) It may cause GI upset.

52. (E) Daily dosing is necessary to maintain therapeutic level.

53. (D) Tween 20 has a high HLB and favors o/w emulsions.

54. (A) Biological half-life does not affect absorption.

55. (C) t 1/2 is equal to 0.693/k in first order kinetics.

56. (B) The parabens slow down mold growth.

57. (E) Propoxyphene (Darvon) is a nonnarcotic analgesic.

58. (B) This is one of the Atlas surfactants.

59. (B) It is an iron containing metalloporphyrin.

60. (C) Air-dried talc imparts a sheen to tablets. Salt is used to polish capsules.

61. (D) It is a nonionic surfactant.

62. (D) 25 x 74.6/1000 = 1.86 g

63. (D) One must count the Na present in the sodium penicillin G.

64. (D) Chloramphenicol is very toxic and tends to cause blood dyscrasias.

65. (D) 87 g/Xg = 1 Eq per 500 ml/0.01 Eq per 500 ml X = 0.87.

66. (C) 74.6 x 0.05 = 3.73

67. (C) Only dialysis can be used. Filtration or centrifugation will not work and salting out or agglutination would damage it.

68. (B) The spectrum is the same, but there is less chance of diarrhea.

69. (C) It is a concentrated form of marijuana.

70. (B) Alcohol causes additive effects.

71. (E) Tetracycline forms complexes with bivalent and trivalent ions.

72. (B) Most are weak acids or weak bases.

73. (B) Hydrolysis occurs to some degree with many drugs.

74. (A) It is an ion exchange resin and replaces potassium with sodium ions.

75. (A) May use different substances to adjust tonicity.

76. (B) It promotes absorption by hydrolizing hyaluronic acid.

77. (C) These are the scientists who developed the equation.

78. (B) This ion product is obtained by adding the pH and pOH.

79. (C) This chelating agent has an affinity for calcium.

80. (C) Rapidly hydrolyzed to acetaminophen.

81. (A) Must exclude moisture primarily.

82. (A) Soap is an anionic surfactant and opposes the action of this cationic detergent.

83. (B) Cold solutions do not penetrate the taste buds as well.

84. (B) This is a slow drip and allows time for distribution.

85. (C) Any prinicple that can be changed to coloring matter.

86. (E) Not w/v. 484 x 0.12 = 58 g

87. (B) They dissolve rapidly under the tongue.
88. (C) The seal on the capsule prevents opening.
89. (A) They give 8-14 hour action.
90. (D) This special device has a metering chamber.
91. (E) The carbonation improves flavor.

92. (A) Hydrolysis produces salicylic acid.

93. (A) These are weak dipole-dipole interactions.

94. (E) It is a histamine inhibitor and acts on H2 receptors.

95. (C) They are absorbed selectively by the liver.

96. (B) The prefix amphi means both or either.

97. (C) Sodium stearate causes solidification of the gel.

98. (C) Silver oxides darken in presence of light.

99. (A) It combines the rate of metabolism and the rate of elimination.

100. (A) Oxidation pathways are less common in vivo.

101. (D) This drug contains a red azo dye.

102. (A) Enzyme pathways differ from animal to animal.

103. (B) Can also use gas sterilization, but not as effective.

104. (C) Its osmotic action reduces edema for short periods.

105. (C) Ethylene oxide gives maximum penetration without destruction of plastic.

106. (A) Syneresis has practical application of removing excess liquid.

107. (C) Original container is very impervious to light.

108. (E) 6 x 100/37 divided by 1.35 = 12 ml

109. (C) 0.5 mg/X mg = 2.2 lb/44 lb (Age not used.)
X = 100 mg (.01 g)

110. (A) Used to relieve gas pains.
111. (C) Nonnarcotic antitussive agents.
112. (B) A surface active agent that absorbs moisture.
113. (E) This drug is a natural bulk-producing laxative.
114. (D) It slows intestinal motility and inhibits peristalsis directly.

115. (E) It is an 18-carbon-atom unsaturated acid.

116. (A) Oxidation occurs readily and produces rancid odor.

117. (C) This is required for laminar flow hoods.

118. (A) The zinc salt is most effective.

119. (D) Imparts a yellowish color.

120. (D) Drug is less available for elimination.

121. (D) This is the commonly used strength.

122. (D) It is a classification system of color.

123. (B) 5 mg/X mg = 2.2 lb/100 kg. X = 227 mg
227/60 = gr approximately

124. (C) These two easily bind drugs.

125. (E) Primary site of action is the loop of Henle.

126. (A) Decrease resorption of sodium and hence increase concentration of lithium.

127. (D) Tetrex is not an antifungal and others are used topically.

128. (A) Over 10% of population experience this. Toxicity is very low.

129. (A) Drug Enforcement Agency (DEA) has replaced BNDD.

130. (D) Needs an acidic pH to be effective. May even be used in combination with acidifiers.

131. (D) Polyvinyl pyrolidone (PVP) forms a soluble complex with iodine (e.g., Isodine).

132. (C) It is a red dye and stains the stool red.

133. (A) Particularly sunburn or steam burns.

134. (B) Aspirin is the most common in accidental poisonings.

135. (C) All tetracyclines can cause irreversible discoloration during tooth-forming years.

136. (B) Potentiation occurs.

137. (D) Benzalkonium in solution rapidly loses its effect.

138. (A) This is true for any oral dosage form.

139. (A) This loop diuretic will continue to act and can produce losses of up to 20 lb per day of fluids.

140. (B) Humans cannot usually hear sound waves over 20 kc.

141. (B) Mucous membrane of the eye could be infected easily.

142. (D) Elastic polymers are used as film coatings.

143. (A) Only weak bonds are formed.

144. (C) Paraaminobenzoic acid used in sunscreens can cause permanent yellow stain on clothing.

145. (B) It is a classical type of first order reaction.

146. (C) It is a measure of oil and water balance in emulsions.

147. (A) Must occur shortly after absorption and prior to biotransformation.

148. (B) Requires no energy, but is very slow.

149. (B) It is used when a hypotonic state is advantageous.

150. (B) Results in formation of insoluble calcium fluoride.

151. (E) They measure relative viscosity compared to water.

152. (B) They have the same mass.

153. (A) They have similar penetrating powers.

154. (B) Because they displace the drug from binding sites.

155. (C) It reacts with bleaches or tints to cause stains.

156. (E) Also a rich source of vitamin D.

157. (D) It is a measure of dispersability or flow of powders.

158. (D) It is directly proportional to the other three factors.

159. (B) Plasma levels are significantly raised in patients using oral contraceptives.

160. (C) Corn or potato starch is used.

161. (D) These fluorinated hydrocarbons are used as propellants in aerosols.

162. (B) Coalescence is followed by creaming or breaking.

163. (A) Bile salts emulsify vitamin A and aid absorption.

164. (C) This is the official description of purity standards.

165. (E) Cationics tend to break complexes.

166. (D) Livers and kidneys commonly become less functional in the elderly.

167. (B) Used in acute attacks of asthma.

168. (B) Several deaths occurred from cyanide poisoning from contaminated capsules.

169. (E) Severe toxicity will result due to aspirin displacement of protein-bound methotrexate.

170. (E) Less than 3.5 kg hardness tablets would cause fragmentation during shipping.

171. (A) This is the primary antidote.

172. (E) Most are foreign proteins.

173. (B) Neutralization occurs.

174. (E) Complications may render them ineffective.

175. (B) It is advisable to give this drug with milk or antacids.

176. (A) Available in crushable ampules for inhalation.

177. (A) Single dose for pinworm.
178. (C) Usual dose for arthritis.
179. (D) Potent antiinflammatory steroid.
180. (E) Medium-spectrum antibiotic.
181. (B) Usual adult dose for epilepsy.

182. (C) It is also called cayenne pepper.

183. (E) Found in many antiperspirant sprays.

184. (C) Shellac is preferred subcoat to prevent erosion during coating.

185. (E) Propranolol produces a hypoglycemic reaction.

186. (D) All others are higher risk categories.

187. (I) A Parke-Davis analgesic.
188. (D) A mercurial diuretic.
189. (A) An MSD psychotropic.
190. (G) A Geigy antiinflammatory.
191. (H) An SKF major tranquilizer.
192. (E) An ultrashort-acting barbiturate by Lilly.
193. (B) An MSD drug used for arthritis.
194. (C) An Abbott tranquilizer.
195. (F) A lilly sedative-hypnotic.
196. (J) An SKF antivertigo drug.

197. (D) The high vapor pressure of nitroglycerin causes this.

198. (C) It makes an alcoholic nauseous if he drinks.

199. (D) Publication in the Federal Register is the only requirement for official notice.

200. (D) Pantopon is a mixture of opium alkaloids.
201. (B) Warfarin is a coumarin derivative.
202. (A) Nortriptylene is a trycyclic antidepressant.
203. (C) It is related to cephalosporin.
204. (E) It is an antimetabolite.

205. (B) Used for asthma attacks in Medihaler.

206. (D) It exerts a drying and peeling action.

207. (A) Adjustment is based on frequency of epileptic seizures.

208. (B) This is a special derivative. Other forms are usually 32 mg or 65 mg.

209. (B) Includes drugs such as heroin, mescaline, LSD.

210. (B) Fermented foods contain tyramine which is toxic in absence or depletion of MAO.

211. (C) The active substance in Marezine.
212. (B) The generic name for Declomycin.
213. (A) Active ingredient.
214. (D) A sustained-release amphetamine.
215. (E) One drug in Ortho-Novum.

216. (C) They are very expensive compared to other dose forms.

217. (B) Inert and soluble so they cause no problems.

218. (B) This dose form contains gas under pressure.

219. (E) $\frac{7.5 \text{ gr}}{0.15 \text{ gr}} = \frac{960}{X}$ minims $\quad X = 6$ minims

220. (A) It darkens on exposure to light.

221. (E) Emetrol is a solution of phosphorylated carbohydrates.

222. (C) Vitamin K is also used to offset effects of indanediones.

223. (B) It chelates copper in vivo.

224. (D) It is used in this form to evacuate the uterus.

225. (A) Terpenes and sesquiterpenes are common.

226. (C) Insoluble compounds form.

227. (A) It is the gummy exudate of unripe capsules of the poppy plant.

228. (E) It is used to soothe sore eyes.

229. (E) All are widely used in clinical trials.

230. (A) Talc is used as a lubricant.

231. (B) Upjohn's antidiarrheal.
232. (E) Abbott's drug for petit mal epilepsy.
233. (A) Abbott's short-acting barbiturate.
234. (C) Abbott's antidandruff drug.
235. (D) Winthrop's nasal decongestant.

236. (C) These are good manufacturing practices.

237. (D) At this point acid/base is 1.0 and log of 1 is 0, so pH = pka.

238. (D) Other methods are useless.

239. (A) Capping commonly occurs with excessive pressure or excessive binder.

240. (E) Friability is measured by rotating tablets in a hollow drum.

241. (C) It effectively reflects light.

242. (D) Peanut oil or cottonseed oil is very popular.

243. (B) This drug permeates cells and paralyzes the parasite.

244. (A) We assume no difference, but hope to disprove null hypothesis.

245. (D) Salicylate analgesics do not compromise its action.

246. (C) It is one of the nitrogen mustards.

247. (B) M is a constant designating slope.

248. (C) $F = 9/5\ c + 32$
$= 9/5\ (78) + 32$
$= 172$

249. (D) A 50:50 dilution is isotonic. It also should be sterile.

250. (C) This dye can stain the hands and underclothing.

251. (A) It is quite acidic and corrosive.

252. (D) This drug actually may cause diarrhea.

253. (A) The smaller the particle, the slower the rate of setting.

254. (D) The Bronsted-Lowry theory is the proton donor-acceptor theory of acids and bases.

255. (E) It is used in topicals to cause sloughing of skin.

256. (E) Very few strains of gonococci are not susceptible.

257. (D) Methyl and propyl paraben are used as preservatives.

258. (A) All of the others are solids.

259. (C) This is used in many cough preparations.

260. (B) Cool air vaporizers are considerably more noisy than the steam type.

261. (D) The name is somewhat misleading, but it is a clay.

262. (E) It is particularly irritating where there are folds in the skin.

263. (E) For this reason, it is commonly dispensed in capsules or highly flavored liquids.

264. (D) This is due to oxidation.

265. (C) It is a popular method to describe odors.

266. (D) It prevents formation of mucus-surrounded gas pockets.

267. (D) It is very effective aginst dermatophytes, particularly tinea infestations.

268. (B) Aluminum chloride is the salt of a strong acid and weak base.

269. (C) It is a tricyclic antidepressant.
270. (A) Particulary effective against tinea versicolor.
271. (D) It is a nonsteroidal agent.
272. (E) It acts directly on the lung.
273. (B) It is a thiazide-type diuretic.

274. (E) The dose is 5 mg per kg of body weight.

275. (B) Para-amino benzoic acid is a good sunscreening agent.

276. (B) Lente is an intermediate-acting insulin combining fast-acting and long-acting forms.

277. (B) Free drug is better for extemporaneous use.
278. (C) This ester is very soluble.
279. (A) This ester has poor stability in acidic vehicles.

280. (C) It is a sulfonamide-type oral diuretic.

281. (C) Salicylates reduce the effectiveness of probenicid.

282. (F) SKF's antipruritic drug.
283. (B) USV nonbarbiturate hypnotic.
284. (D) Lilly's nonbarbiturate hypnotic.
285. (A) Ciba's topical antifungal agent.
286. (G) Roche's minor tranquilizer.
287. (E) Abbott's nonbarbiturate hypnotic.
288. (C) Pfizer's broad-spectrum antibiotic.

289. (E) Ideal potassium nutrient level.

290. (D) Abbott's matrix-type sustained-release tablet.
291. (B) Winthrop's quick-dissolving tablet.
292. (A) Metered dose aerosol form.
293. (E) Schering's distinctively colored tablets.
294. (C) Abbott's brand of disposable syringe.

295. (B) Children's cough syrup with low concentration of ipecac for expectorant action.

296. (B) Unstable at high pH.

297. (D) This antianginal agent is used in ointment form.

298. (B) This drug inhibits fibrinolysis.

299. (C) Other strengths would be excessive.

300. (D) Damage to retina was seen in animal studies by the FDA.

301. (B) Needs about 30% water present for solvent action.

302. (B) Seldom used because of this.

303. (C) Drug is poorly absorbed by other routes.

304. (A) Pyridoxine is the synonym for B_6.

305. (A) Chloromycetin is produced by Streptomyces venezuelae.
306. (E) Erythromycin is produced by Streptomyces erythreus.
307. (D) Vancomycin is produced by Streptomyces orientalis.
308. (B) Novobiocin is produced by Streptomyces niveus.
309. (C) Streptomycin is produced by Streptomyces griseus.

310. (B) This will completely screen burning rays of the sun.

311. (I) SKF's sustained-release OTC cold preparation.
312. (G) OTC suspension to coat the stomach and reduce acidity.
313. (B) An OTC cough preparation containing cetamium.
314. (E) OTC antiemetic that is particularly effective for motion sickness.
315. (C) OTC product containing calamine and a local anesthetic to reduce itching.
316. (A) OTC nontherapeutic vitamin capsule.
317. (D) Contains kaolin and pectin.
318. (J) Mild laxative action.
319. (F) Tends to shrink hemorrhoids and provide local anesthetic action.
320. (H) In the form of a tincture to paint onto minor wounds.

321. (C) It combines a short- and an intermediate-acting barbiturate for quick onset and longer action.

322. (C) It is used to treat yeast and fungus infestations in an ophthalmic suspension.

323. (C) Pink color is due primarily to red Fe_2O_3.

324. (E) It is a fluorinated hydrocarbon gas.
325. (D) It is a reducing agent that retards oxidation.
326. (C) It is a naturally occurring dye.
327. (A) It imparts a fruity flavor.
328. (F) This gum forms viscous preparations.
329. (B) This is vaseline.
330. (I) It is a solvent in many pharmaceuticals.
331. (H) It is a common diluent in tablets and capsules.
332. (K) This is cocoa butter that melts at body temperature.
333. (G) It is an effective binder which also improves disintegration.
334. (L) This substance improves flow properties and reduces sticking.
335. (J) It is used to adjust pH and buffer capacity.

336. (C) 473 g x 8 x 1.25 = 4730

337. (C) Equivalent in minims for a fluid dram.
338. (E) Equivalent in ml for a pint (29.57 x 16).
339. (F) Equivalent in minims of 1 ml.
340. (A) Equivalent in mg of 1 grain (usually rounded off to 65 mg).
341. (B) 16 oz x 8 = 128 fl oz
342. (D) Weight of 1 dram in grains.
343. (G) Weight of an avoirdupois pound in grams.

344. (D) Reduces swelling in membrane.
345. (E) Acts on the cough center in the medulla.
346. (C) Keeps the throat moist.
347. (A) Commonly used for these purposes.
348. (B) Stimulates breakup of phlegm.

349. (E) Tinctures are alcoholic solutions of vegetable, animal or chemical substances and are usually 5-20% in strength.

350. (E) Vitamin K is necessary for formation of prothrombin.

351. (D) Cobalt is an element in the chemical structure.

352. (A) This is an ophthalmic solution of phenylephrine.
353. (E) This is a vaginal insert.
354. (C) A solution for nebulization.
355. (B) Much too toxic for any other route.
356. (D) Should never be given IV.

357. (C) It is used as a stabilizer (antioxidant).
358. (D) It is used to enhance emulsification and incorporation.
359. (B) Used as a denaturant in many rubbing alcohols.
360. (E) This substance imparts the enteric coating activity.
361. (A) It is a critical ingredient to make collodion.

362. (A) The dose is similar regardless of route.
363. (D) This is the usual strength given every four hours.
364. (B) This is the common strength as an analgesic.
365. (C) This vitamin is given in international units.
366. (E) This oral anthelmintic is adjusted based on body weight.

367. (H) Dosage is increased until side effects occur.
368. (G) Applied to teeth in this strength.
369. (F) This is the normal maintenance dose.
370. (J) This is the analeptic dose
371. (I) This is the daily dietary requirement.

372. (F) It is a potent nonnarcotic analgesic without addicting properties.
373. (G) It is an internal drug used to reduce itching.
374. (H) It is a nonsalicylate and nonsteroid drug used to treat arthritis.
375. (K) It was originally designed as treatment for myasthenia, but is used more for diagnosis.
376. (C) It is a nonnarcotic, antihistaminic cough preparation.
377. (A) It was the first effective antihistamine and is still widely used.
378. (I) It is a phenothiazine derivative originally intended as a tranquilizer.
379. (E) It is methocarbamol and is widely used for indirect muscle relaxation.
380. (B) Serotonin blocker used as a prophylactic against migraine or to reduce intensity of attacks.
381. (M) It is used mainly to treat petit mal epilepsy.
382. (L) It is an oral diuretic of the thiazide type.
383. (J) It got its name because it is used to elevate the mood.
384. (D) Used mainly for vaginal fungal infestations. Inserted with applicator.

385. (C) It is a concentrated form of Kaopectate.
386. (D) Over-the-counter mild hypnotic.
387. (G) Has excellent expectorant action.
388. (H) Flavored, low-calorie powder or liquid.
389. (F) Jelly containing a local anesthetic.
390. (L) It is also a buffer, to reduce acid rebound.
391. (A) It provides heat and counterirritant action.
392. (I) It is particularly useful for sunburn.
393. (K) Shrinks hemorrhoids and relieves discomfort.
394. (B) It is adjusted to tonicity and pH of eye fluids.
395. (M) Contains zirconium and benadryl.
396. (J) It contains chondrus which is a bulk producer.
397. (E) It is used as an aspirin substitute.

398. (C) Carbowax is merely a trade name used for this group.

399. (A) It is a high molecular weight polymer that is miscible with organic solvents and some oils.

400. (F) $\bar{c}$ is an abbreviation for the latin word *cum.*
401. (H) Usually translated as tablespoonful.
402. (G) Latin word *pulveres* means powder.
403. (A) Also translated as once an hour.
404. (B) Latin is *secundum artem.*
405. (J) Latin word for make is *fiat.*
406. (D) M. is abbreviation for *misce* (to mix).
407. (C) Latin *ante cibum* means before meals.
408. (L) Abbreviation for Latin phrase *si opus sit.*
409. (E) Literally means aerated water, but is used to denote carbonation.
410. (M) Literally translated "as dictated."
411. (I) *Gutta* is Latin word for drop.
412. (N) Also used to mean initial order as in a "stat order"
413. (K) Also used to denote dusting powders.

414. (B) Abbreviation for Latin *oculo sinistre.*
415. (E) Combination of Latin abbreviation.
416. (J) Also may be translated "as needed."
417. (A) *Oculo dextro* means right eye. Sometimes confused with translation "everyday."
418. (C) Literally means small spoonful which is a teaspoonful.
419. (F) Latin words are *oculo utro.*
420. (G) Literally means give of such doses to number four.
421. (D) Also may be translated as alternate days.
422. (I) Literally means "in the manner prescribed."
423. (H) Latin word is *sine.*

424. (B) $6.0 - 5.6 = 0.4$
Antilog of 0.4 is 2.5
Since 6 was added it must be subtracted in the exponent.

425. (A) Lacrimal fluid has a slightly acidic pH.

426. (D) Desenex contains undecylenic acid which has antifungal activity.
427. (A) Paradione is one of Abbott's antiepileptic agents
428. (F) Dopar is Eaton's brand of L-Dopa.
429. (B) Coumadin is Endo's brand of warfarin.
430. (I) Hedulin is Merrell's brand of phenindione.
431. (C) Compazine is SKF's brand of prochlorperazine.
432. (E) Fungizone is Squibb's brand of amphotericin B.
433. (K) Gantrisin is Roche's brand of sulfisoxazole.
434. (G) Neutrapen is a brand name for the enzyme penicillinase which is used as an antidote for penicillin.
435. (H) Serpasil is a Ciba brand of reserpine.
436. (J) Bristol's trade name for ampicillin.
437. (L) Santyl is Knoll's brand name for the enzyme collagenase.

438. (E) $1/X = 200/120$ $\quad X = 0.6$ g
$5 \text{ g}/0.6 \text{ g} = 100 \text{ ml}/X \text{ ml}$ $\quad X = 12$ ml

439. (C) $28.4 \text{ g} + 29.6 \text{ g} = 58 \text{ g}$
$28.4 \text{ g}/X = 58 \text{ g}/100$ $\quad X = 48.6\%$

440. (A) This drug may mask symptoms of infection.

441. (C) $F = 9/5\,(-12^\circ) + 32$
$= 10.4^\circ$

442. (A) A tablespoon is about one-half ounce or 15 ml.

443. (A) Vibramycin is Pfizer's brand name for doxycycline.
444. (B) Cotazym is Organon's trade name for pancreolipase.
445. (M) Rondomycin is a trade name for methacycline which is a derivative of oxytetracycline.
446. (I) Tegretol is the brand name (Geigy) for carbamazepine used for trigeminal neuralgia.
447. (O) Diazepam is the generic name for Valium (Roche).
448. (G) Skelaxin is Robins' brand name for metaxolone.
449. (C) Banthine is Searle's brand of methantheline.
450. (N) Furacin is Eaton's name for nitrofurazone.
451. (J) Squibb's trade name for triamcinolone.
452. (H) Squibb's brand of procainamide.
453. (F) Ciba's trade name for glutethimide.

454. (E) Lilly's brand name for thiamine of B_1.
455. (K) Ilotycin is Lilly's brand of erythromycin.
456. (D) Geigy's brand name for chlorthalidone.
457. (E) See answer #454.

458. (B) Reinfection is likely if the drug is used for less than 10 days.

459. (B) Must use tests that don't involve acid precipitation as end point.

460. (A) Kaolin is an excellent absorbent for toxins causing diarrhea.

461. (D) Dolophine is Lilly's trade name for methadone.

462. (E) This drug may precipitate acute attacks of psoriasis.

463. (A) Makes plaque on teeth more visible.

464. (E) Apomorphine is a synthetic analog of morphine.

465. (C) Disulfiram inhibits aldehyde dehydrogenase.

466. (D) Carbidopa acts only to slow destruction of levodopa.

467. (E) It is a cream used for cleansing and antiseptic value.

468. (C) This is Mayer's reagent.

469. (D) This drug interaction is marked and even extends to other antipsychotic agents.

470. (B) Only the salts are very water soluble.

471. (B) Barrier creams prevent rhus toxin from reaching the skin or spreading.

472. (B) Minimizes interactions with the container.

473. (C) It releases undecylenic acid to combat fungus.

474. (C) Enzymes in fungus break down triacetin to release acetic acid.

475. (A) Tolnaftate is very effective in extremely small doses.

476. (B) It slows down decarboxylation.

477. (A) It is the alcohol obtained from wool fat.

478. (E) Simethicone has coating action and the others are mild alkalinizers.

479. (D) It is similar to amikacin.

480. (B) It may ruin soft contact lenses.

481. (A) OTC analgesic with anticramping properties.

482. (B) It is absorbed and places a charge on suspended particles to prevent floculation.

483. (B) It is selenium sulfide.

484. (C) Xerostomia is severe dryness of the mouth.

485. (E) Protamine zinc insulin is slowly released and longer acting.

486. (A) It contains carbamide peroxide which releases oxygen.

487. (C) They vary in molecular weight and are prepared by polymerization.

488. (J) Freon II is a fluorinated hydrocarbon used as a propellant.
489. (F) Acacia is a plant gum.
490. (E) Pyrvinium pamoate is a red cyanine dye used for pinworms.
491. (G) Emetrol is a mixture of phosphorylated carbohydrates.

492. (D) The Stormer is a type of viscosimeter.
493. (A) The Ainsworth is a type of analytical balance.
494. (B) DuBosc developed the original colorimeter.
495. (C) The Strong-Cobb is the most widely used type of hardness tester for tablets.
496. (H) The Patterson-Kelly is the so-called V shell or twin shell blender.
497. (I) The Fitzpatrick-type mill is widely used.

498. (A) Thioglycollates are less irritating to skin.

499. (D)

95	70	70	X	
0				X = 368 ml
		25		
		95	500	

500. (E) Gums are more water soluble.

501. (D) 14 minus 11 = 3

502. (E) The continental method is used for extemporaneous preparation of emulsions.
503. (C) Granulation is used to prepare powdered materials to flow better for tableting.
504. (D) The freezing point depression method is used to calculate the amount of NaCl or other additives.
505. (B) The Van Slyke equation is used to determine buffer capacity.
506. (A) Ideal flow is Newtonian flow.

507. (B) Geigy's anticonvulsant.
508. (I) Fisons' antiasthmatic inhalant.
509. (F) Parke Davis antihyperlipidemic.
510. (J) Winthrop's vasoconstrictor.
511. (E) Flint's thyroid hormone.
512. (A) Ciba's adrenal steroid inhibitor.
513. (C) One of Schering's glucocorticoids.
514. (D) Schering's antifungal.
515. (G) Winthrop's analgesic.
516. (H) Roerig's antianxiety agent.

517. (E) It is a phenothiazine derivative.

518. (C) It is a nonirritating form of iodine.

519. (B) Because they are pressurized containers which could explode.

520. (A) Should not be frozen.

521. (B) 1/5 x 30 = 6 ml

522. (C) It interferes with impulse transmission from sympathetic nerves to the cardiovascular system.

523. (D) It is a gold compound used for adjunctive treatment of early active rheumatoid arthritis.

524. (E) Loxapine is an antipsychotic, but not a phenothiazene.

525. (B) Lower concentrations are not anesthetic and higher concentrations are unnecessary.

526. (E) It absorbs water readily and keeps moisture in.

527. (C) Controls convulsions by blocking neuromuscular response.

528. (B) They potentiate the action of anticoagulants markedly.

529. (B) It is lethal to amoeba that cause dysentery.

530. (C) The other types melt to release drug.

531. (E) Sodium sulfacetamide is found in many eye solutions and ointments.

532. (B) It releases hydrogen peroxide.

533. (C) The National Association of Boards of Pharmacy handles reciprocity.

534. (B) This includes prescription and inventory data.

535. (A) Prolongs the action and prevents absorption.

536. (D) This dye colors the urine reddish-orange.

537. (B) Surfactants with very high HLB are most useful to form micelles.

538. (C) Tweens are the atlas group of polysorbates.

539. (C) Used to calm the patient who is hyperexcitable.

540. (D) It is an oxidized cellulose that is later absorbable.

541. (A) It has antipruritic activity.

542. (B) This means it may only be used for research or testing.

543. (A) It creates an opaque medium for x-ray.

544. (C) The American Council on Pharmaceutical Education accredits all schools.

545. (D) This measures copper sulfate reduction.
546. (B) Used to estimate amount of urea nitrogen in whole blood.
547. (A) Detects presence of occult blood in urine or feces.
548. (C) Detects presence of leukocytes in the urine
549. (E) These are multiple test coated strips.
550. (F) Tablets are dissolved and show color in presence of bilirubin.

551. (D) It has a direct but mild action on the CTZ.

552. (B) Patient tends to become very sensitive to bright light.

553. (A) It is used for actue attacks of gout.

554. (A) The diuretic action of digitalis tends to deplete potassium.

555. (A) Digitalis does not act in this way.

556. (B) Gives same hypotensive effect as alcohol does with Antabuse.

557. (B) This drug is poorly absorbed orally and is not useful during acute attacks.

558. (B) This drug will thus cause constipation.

559. (C) It is used in emergencies to overcome shock.
560. (A) It is a sympathomimetic alkaloid.
561. (B) A thiazide-type diuretic.
562. (E) A loop diuretic.
563. (D) It is used primarily for ventricular fibrillation.

564. (C) It is used to treat supraventricular tachycardia.
565. (B) It inhibits the CTZ in the medulla.
566. (E) This is a broad-spectrum agent.
567. (D) It is used to treat lead poisoning primarily.
568. (A) It is used to treat inflammation of musculoskeletal or soft tissue.

569. (C) Breaks down mucus and aids in its elimination from respiratory tract.

570. (A) Anticholinergics are not useful in treating this disease.

571. (E) It interferes with synthesis of lymph-cell macromolecules and alkylates DNA.

572. (E) Digitalis poisoning is fairly common, but tolerance, dependence or addiction is not common.

573. (D) Newer drug that is more effective than salicylates or corticosteroids.
574. (A) Very potent and can even cause paralysis of muscles in high doses.
575. (E) Potent diuretic action even when given orally.
576. (B) Essential for formation of RBC.
577. (C) Potent antihypertensive; also has major tranquilizer activity.

578. (A) Barbiturates depress respiration in high doses.

579. (A) Reduces flow of impulses to conscious centers.

580. (B) Rapid convulsions occur and tax the respiratory center.

581. (D) Must be taken early in the attack. Constricts the blood vessels and relieves symptoms.
582. (C) Usually administered by inhalation and acts quickly.
583. (B) Used to treat severe hypotension associated with shock.
584. (A) This is an enzyme which reduces inflammation in injuries.
585. (E) Used mainly to relieve itching in urticaria.

586. (C) Results in stimulation and convulsions.

587. (C) It acts by preventing fibrinolysis.

588. (B) Marked potentiation occurs if calcium levels are high.

589. (B) Probably due to effects on lungs.

590. (A) Dosage is regularly adjusted upward if attacks occur frequently.

591. (A) Loss of appetite and distress are usually the first visible signs.

592. (C) Prevents conversion to organic form and thus prevents uptake.

593. (A) This is a cholinergic effect.

594. (C) Naqua is trichlormeththiazide—a thiazide diuretic.
595. (E) Velban is an alkylating agent used to treat carcinomas.
596. (B) Librium and Equanil are both minor tranquilizers.
597. (A) Sansert is a prophylactic drug for migraine.
598. (B) See answer # 596.
599. (C) See answer # 594. Chlorothiazide is another thiazide diuretic.
600. (D) Broad-spectrum antihistaminic.

601. (B) Many patients are allergic to this drug.
602. (C) Can be delayed by massaging the gums frequently.
603. (D) This drug is contraindicated for children during the toothforming years.
604. (A) Ringing in the ears is a common side effect with this drug.

605. (D) If arrest occurs, it is due to asystole.

606. (D) It is a selective adrenergic used for treatment of asthma.

607. (B) BAL is also used for poisoning by other heavy metals.

608. (B) May cause temporary or permanent hearing damage.

609. (C) It is very useful when prompt or urgent decrease of diastolic pressure is required.

610. (D) The weakened muscles are more susceptible to paralysis.

611. (A) Oxidized prior to excretion by the kidneys primarily.

612. (D) Polycarbophil restores normal moisture levels in either constipation or diarrhea.

613. (E) This is due to the fact that it is metabolized to formic acid and formaldehyde.

614. (B) See answer # 613.

615. (C) This antibiotic agent has practically no effect on other carcinomas.

616. (E) It causes a change in the metabolism of carbohydrates, proteins and fats.

617. (B) It must be administered by inhalation for this reason.

618. (C) Vitamin K is a specific antidote for the coumarins and indanediones.

619. (B) The other agents are used primarily for bone marrow carcinomas or lymphatic carcinomas.

620. (D) Alternate-day therapy for other conditions has not been highly successful.

621. (D) It stimulates production of this enzyme.

622. (A) It is not well absorbed.

623. (B) The other concentrations are excessive for IV use.

624 (C) Central effects of local anesthetics are undesirable.

625. (E) It is a strongly alkaline organic amine.

626. (A) It may even increase both values slightly.

627. (A) Usually months or years pass before this type of asthmatic develops aspirin tolerance.

628. (E) This is responsible for its emetic action.

629. (D) Seldom used to treat amebiasis even though it has amebicidal activity, because of its side effect of causing emesis.

630. (A) It sensitizes the myocardium to all catecholamines.

631. (C) It directly antagonizes action of curare.

632. (E) It forms an insoluble complex and ties up lead.

633. (B) Dosage is adjusted based on prothrombin time.

634. (C) Receptor is right at the muscle.

635. (E) It provides a combination of diuretic and antihypertensive action.

636. (D) Ganglionic blockers decrease all secretions in general.

637. (C) This drug is a benzodiazepine derivative.

638. (D) It is a specific B_2 stimulant with practically no effects on other receptors.

639. (E) This estrogenic substance has been used somewhat successfully arresting this type of carcinoma.

640. (A) It is one of the fluorinated hydrocarbon-type general inhalation anesthetics.

641. (E) The other drugs act too slowly to be used for acute attacks.

642. (B) Asphyxiation is due to the inability of the hemo globin to carry oxygen.

643. (D) It is particularly effective in treating the rickett-sial infection typhoid fever.

644. (C) Its toxicity to bone marrow is minimal, but it is unusually toxic to the skin and lungs.

645. (D) This is commonly used to adjust dosage.

646. (A) This cholinergic agnet is used primarily to treat glaucoma. It causes marked miosis.

647. (C) The causative organism is a group A hemolytic streptococcus.

648. (E) It is available in an aerosol for reversible ob-structive airway conditions.

649. (B) Atropine is more effective against muscarinic effects.

650. (D) This is a gonadotropic hormone.

651. (A) The conjugation is primarily by acetylation.

652. (D) It has fewer side effects but diminishes secretions.

653. (A) Fungi secrete an enzyme that breaks down the triacetin.

654. (B) It is faster acting than warfarin which is the only other anticoagulant listed here.

655. (C) It is stable and well absorbed from the GI tract.

656. (B) 100 mg of Demerol versus 10-12 mg of morphine.

657. (D) Used primarily in relapsing vivax malaria for this reason.

658. (D) This is an effective antifungal agent for candida infestations.

659. (B) It is an oral hypoglycemic agent.

660. (A) There is decreased resistance to infection and inability to localize infection.

661. (A) All of the others block the sympathetic nervous system, and are not indicated in emergency treatment of hypertensive crisis.

662. (C) It is a narcotic and has significant addicting properties.

663. (A) The disease is characterized by low levels of brain dopamine.

664. (A) Estrogens increase incidence and the others listed have no effect.

665. (B) Overdoses paralyze all muscles. This is a curare derivative.

666. (D) Antihistamines do not change histamine levels. It is competitive inhibition that makes them effective.

667. (D) Acts directly to depress the cough center in the medulla.

668. (D) Pralidoxime is an emergency antidote.

669. (D) Most iron salts blacken the stool.

670. (E) They exert no action on the vestibular apparatus. Their primary action is directly on the CTZ.

671. (C) Medullary paralysis can occur with overdoses.

672. (D) It is used mainly for controlling capillary leakage.

673. (E) It directly relaxes vascular smooth muscle.

674. (C) The acetate is only slightly soluble and gives prolonged action.

675. (C) It is structurally similar to morphine derivatives and has some agonistic activity.

676. (D) It is an effective uterine relaxant.

677. (C) This is due to interference with peristalsis.

678. (A) It interferes with uric acid synthesis and is a good prophylactic agent to prevent gout.

679. (D) It increases norepinephrine levels, but interfers with nerve impulse transmission to the cardiovascular system.

680. (A) Occurs only if absorption takes place.

681. (C) Due to shallow respiration caused by medullary depression.

682. (C) This antifungal agent is very effective.

683. (E) All of the listed actions are characteristic of this compound.

684. (C) This drug is also useful in treating hypertension.

685. (B) This drug lowers levels of all fats, and not just cholesterol.

686. (B) It is strongly bacteriocidal to this bacillus.

687. (D) Act by competitive inhibition in the mucosa.
688. (C) Act directly on the cough center of the medulla.
689. (A) Acts in lower CNS as an antidepressant.
690 (E) Build up moisture.
691. (B) Block these receptors and prevent release of dopamine.

692. (E) Protects L-Dopa to increase effectiveness.
693. (D) Passes blood-brain barrier and is converted.
694. (B) It is a nondepolarizing blocker.
695. (C) Acts peripherally to reduce norepinephrine levels.
696. (A) It slows motility and is useful in treating diarrhea.

697. (E) This is kaolin, pectin and opium alkaloid.
698. (C) This is a direct-acting muscle relaxant.
699. (B) It is a tricyclic antidepressant.
700. (D) It is an oral antidiabetic.
701. (A) It is used to treat ulcers.

702. (B) This drug should be given with food to prevent this effect.
703. (E) All sulfonamides have a tendency to produce allergic reactions.
704. (D) Severe allergic responses are fairly common with penicillins.
705. (A) It is preferable to take Sinutabs with coffee or other stimulant beverages for this reason.
706. (C) Ringing in the ears is a common side effect of this drug.

707. (A) It is a specific antagonist to curare.

708. (B) This drug suppresses neuromuscular transmission.
709. (D) The discoloration is temporary and causes no symptoms or harm.
710. (E) This is due to erythrocytes which are deficient in glucose-6-phosphate dehydrogenase.
711. (C) Often has to be given IM because of this.
712. (A) Few problems if used in therapeutic dosage.

713. (B) Marked effect on respiration. This drug has a relatively low margin of safety.
714. (C) Used mainly for dental surgery.
715. (D) It is the most potent of the inhalation anesthetics.
716. (E) Almost never used because of its deficiencies.
717. (A) Induction is rapid and it produces less secretions than many of the inhalation anesthetics.

718. (E) Does not condition barbituric acid nucleus.
719. (D) Over 8 hours duration.
720. (C) Slow onset and acts for up to 6 hours.
721. (B) Acts for about 4 hours.
722. (A) Effect lasts for less than 1 hour. Used mainly as preanesthetic or anesthetic.

723. (C) Oral contraceptives may cause thromboembolitis.
724. (A) This is an adrenal steroid inhibitor.
725. (D) This drug can induce or worsen aplastic anemia.
726. (E) A side effect is potent uterine stimulation.
727. (B) This drug is excreted largely by the lungs.

728. D) Deficiency of B_1 produces beriberi.

729. (A) Frequently given in suppository form for long action.

730. (D) It is an antithyroid compound which interferes with iodine uptake.

731. C) All of the alkylating antineoplastic agents depress WBC.
732. (C) Does this by inducing prolonged contractions of the uterus. Best of ergot alkaloids for this use.
733. (D) This a rather broad-spectrum anthelminthic.
734. (E) This drug is an antimetabolite used to treat carcinomas.
735. (A) It is one of the coumarin group which blocks or slows prothrombin synthesis.
736. (B) It is an analog of chlorpheniramine and combines antihistaminic effect with a marked sedative side effect.

737. (B) Theophylline decreases phenytoin levels markedly.
738. (A) Propoxyphene increases blood levels of carbamazepine.
739. (C) Action of colchicine is inhibited by these agents.
740. (E) Isoniazid impairs clearance and increases the half-life.
741. (D) Potassium ion antagonizes the action of pancuronium.

742. (E) This antimalarial causes yellow pigmentation of the skin which disappears when the drug is discontinued.

743. (D) Codeine has weaker analgesic properties than many of the other alkaloids.
744. (E) There is no antagonism of papaverine by the narcotic antagonist nalophine.
745. (B) Antispasmodic activity is mild
746. (A) The addicting properties of methadone are much milder than other derivatives.
747. (C) This the principal alkaloid of the opium plant.

748. (E) It is a glucocorticoid.

749. (D) This is a combintion of diampterine and hydrochlorothiazide.
750. (C) Combination of aspirin, phenacetin, caffeine, and butabital.
751. (B) This is tolnaftate, which is a topical antifungal.
752. (E) This is a strong choline esterase inhibitor.
753. (A) This is an antianxiety agent with excellent muscle relaxant properties.

754. (D) Cardiovascular side effects are enhanced.

755. (C) It is a specific antagonist of aldosterone.

756. (B) It has no effect on force of heart muscle.

757. (A) Increased renal clearance would reduce its effects.

758. (D) Phenothiazines interfere with uptake of guanethidine.

805. (F) This contains blood-clotting factors.
806. (B) This is a prostaglandin.
807. (A) This decreases extraction of fatty acids.
808. (D) This is a general CNS depressant.
809. (I) This is used primarily to treat petit mal epilepsy.
810. (H) This is a hydrophilic colloid used to increase bulk.
811. (G) This substance increases sloughing of lesions.

812. (B) Similar in structure and exhibits competitive inhibition.
813. (C) Allergic responses are mainly rashes.
814. (D) Only agent that will eliminate both.
815. (A) Should not be given parenterally.
816. (F) Has replaced streptomycin to a great degree.
817. (E) Have practically eradicated this disease.

818. (B) It comes from the vinca rosea plant.
819. (A) It is an enzyme substance used in lymphocytic leukemias.
820. (E) It mainly affects bone marrow.
821. (D) It interferes with RNA and DNA formation or utilization.
822. (C) Produces severe nausea with each dose.

823. (C) This is an oral hypoglycemic used for adult-onset diabetes.
824. (D) This antihistamine alleviates symptoms.
825. (B) Suppository form of this drug is preferred.
826. (F) Ergot alkaloids relieve symptoms if given early in attack.
827. (E) Primarily used for grand mal type of seizure or status epilepticus.
828. (A) Prophylactic to cut down on synthesis or uric acid.
829. (G) Phenobarbital is a short-acting barbiturate.
830. (H) Dieting is preferable because of side effects and danger of abuse.

831. (C) Both are histamine antagonists.
832. (D) Both are mild diuretics.
833. (A) Both are loop diuretics.
834. (B) Both are oral hypoglycemics.
835. (F) Both are antacids.
836. (E) Both are analgesics.
837. (G) Both are calcium channel blockers.

838. (B) It has stimulant action on CNS.

839. (B) It is reflectant to light and blocks harmful rays.

840. (C) Oxidation occurs to form this.
841. (E) Enzyme-mediated.
842. (J) No detoxication necessary
843. (A) Oxidation is slow which accounts for long half-life.
844. (F) This is the principal metabolite.
845. (G) Enzyme breaks down this amine.
846. (H) All sulfonamides are excreted mainly as acetyl derivatives.
847. (B) Detoxication is mobilized by glucuronides.
848. (D) Forms a uric acid derivative.
849. (I) Phenothiazines form sulfoxides.

850. (B) Most useful for this type of seizure or status epelipticus.
851. (E) Alternate drug for petit mal.
852. (A) Far more toxic than others. It causes direct organ toxicity.
853. (F) Not seen with other CNS drugs.
854. (D) Potentiation is marked.
855. (C) This is an analeptic agent and is not at all useful in epilepsies.

856. (E) This is ethylenediamine-tetraacetic acid and is only useful as salt.
857. (G) This folic acid antagonist is used as an anti-neoplastic.
858. (B) Used to combat poisoning by heavy metals.
859. (D) At postganglionic sites in sympathetic nervous system.
860. (H) Reverses effects of cyanide poisoning.
861. (A) Competes for receptor sites.
862. (J) Useful for chronic alcoholism.
863. (C) Its name denotes its action
864. (F) It acts as a mild diuretic for this reason.
865. (I) DFP is an anticholinergic agent.

866. (C) Potent antihypertensive action.
867. (D) All mercurial diuretics cause inflammation of gums.
868. (A) Decreases normal peristalsis.

869. (E) This is a phenothiazine compound.
870. (F) This may be a useful side effect, if patient has motion sickness.

871. (A) It acts as an obligatory osmotic diuretic.
872. (C) It inhibits synthesis of thyroid hormone.
873. (B) It is used to prevent or treat ventricular fibrillation.
874. (D) It is a peripheral vasodilator.
875. (E) It lowers serum triglyceride levels.

876. (E) This occurs only occasionally, but may be a problem with diabetics.

877. (D) Other dibenzazepines do not exert their effects for weeks.

878. (C) The other agents are not primarily antitubercular.

879. (D) Adds to hyperexcitability of hyperthyroid patient.

880. (B) Must be given by injection. Other statements are untrue.

881. (E) All of the statements are false.

882. (D) Effective in treating some acute lymphocytic anemias.

883. (A) It raises blood pressure and increases circulation rapidly.

884. (C) Only discontinuation is indicated. Tolerance reverses after withdrawal.

885. (A) Primary site is in distal tubule just beyond loop of Henle.

886. (A) It is a potent oral agent.

887. (D) They do not counteract increased gastric secretion.

888. (E) Bradykinin has no effect on bronchioles.

889. (C) It prevents biotransformation of catecholamines.

890. (A) It has a markedly shorter duration of action, but does depress respiration and dosage adjustment is a problem.

891. (E) It is used mainly for the GI tract, however.

892. (B) The major use of Regitine is for that purpose.

893. (D) It relaxes the uterus.

894. (D) It is also used for parathione poisoning because it reverses its action.

895. (E) These drugs are long acting.

896. (B) Diuretics are used first, because hypertension is triggered by salt retention.

897. (B) This drug prolongs the QT interval.

898. (A) Has antiinflammatory and analgesic activity.

899. (E) Levodopa can cross the blood-brain barrier and dopamine cannot.

900. (C) An immunosuppressive agent which has low toxicity.

901. (D) It is an antiviral agent.

902. (E) Severe allergic reactions are not uncommon.

903. (A) Toxin produces local reaction unless neutralized by circulating antitoxin.

904. (E) Believed to inhibit viral replication.

905. (D) Drug of choice for susceptible strains of P. aeruginosa.

906. (E) Live attenuated virus with longer period of immunity and does require special labeling.

907. (A) Requires elimination of barbiturate or upward adjustment of griseofulvin dosage.

908. (C) Fixed by complement to form bacteriocidal defense.
909. (D) Mobilize body defenses against bacteria.
910. (E) Heat-labile groups.
911. (B) Can act without presence of complement to agglutinate bacteria.
912. (A) Usually used in vitro.

913. (B) This is a description of the vaccine.

914. (C) This is a killed virus, and this is to ensure that it is.

915. (D) The methods are used alone or in combination to ensure attenuation.

916. (A) Unnecessary, because killed organisms are just as effective.

917. (D) It is a polyvalent antivenom which is useful for all of these and others.

918. (C) The common name is german measles.

919. (E) Only controls toxin until it becomes fixed onto nervous tissue.

920. (D) Requires fast action before fixation on nervous tissue.

921. (C) Antibody levels persist for 6-7 years.

922. (B) Made from globulin fraction of animal sera.

923. (A) Usually listed as units based on MLD.

924. (D) There is up to a 40% incidence of this side effect.

925. (D) The other drugs are antifungal agents and have little or no effect on bacteria.

926. (D) It loses its effectiveness.

927. (E) Original outbreaks were in forest country.

928. (B) Usually rises in afternoon and falls at night.

929. (A) Usual carrier.

930. (A) Got its name from rise and fall.

931. (E) Spherical eosinophilic cell inclusions found only in rabies.

932. (A) Also carried by the rabbit louse.

933. (E) Penicillin is most effective on rapidly growing microorganisms.

934. (A) Marked nausea, vomiting and diarrhea cause this.

935. (A) Seldom involves throat or tonsils in children.

936. (C) Due to formation of a speudomembrane.

937. (A) The causative organism is P. pestis.

938. (A) Exotoxins are treated with formaldehyde and then purified.

939. (D) These are reddened areas of the buccal mucosa.

940. (A) It is an ampicillin derivative.

941. (E) This agent is effective against whipworm, hookworm, trichinosis and Strongyloides.

942. (E) This organism will not ferment lactose or sucrose.

943. (B) FDA launched a massive program a few years ago to reduce sources of salmonella contamination in both foods and drugs.

944. (D) However, some active cases do not give a positive test.

945. (E) Usually caused by Tricophyton group of fungi or Epidermophyton floccosum.

946. (A) Used only where other penicillins fail because of rapid development of resistant strains.

947. (B) Should be reserved for serious infections where other agents fail.

948. (C) It is usually given on small cubes of sugar.

949. (C) This yields energy.

950. (B) This is one of the enterococcus organisms associated with these conditions.

951 (D) Man is the only natural host for whom meningococci are pathogenic.

952. (A) Rats, rabbits, hares and muskrats in particular.

953. (C) It produces less marked effect on GI system in general.

954. (D) Very effective when used in combination with other agents.

955. (C) Fever is lower in AM and tends to peak in late afternoon or early evening.

956. (B) Gives false-positive with Clinitest or Benedict's.

957. (B) They are anaerobic gram-positive rods, and spore forms are very resistant to heat.

958. (A) Causative rickettsia is R. prowazekii.

959. (D) It is particularly effective in vaginal moniliasis.

960. (C) Changes it chemically to make it permanent.

961. (D) The methods listed in A, B, and C will not kill most spores.

962. (E) It has a similar spectrum, but is a beta-lactam.

963. (E) It is usually only 2-3 weeks, but may be much longer.

964. (E) The term may be defined in either way.

965. (E) Kaolin reduces absorption of clindamycin.

966. (D) The other answers list the four growth phases.

967. (A) Septic sore throat is caused by hemolytic streptococci.

968. (D) A betalactam antibiotic closely related to the cephalosporins.

969 (B) It is used to treat inflammations caused by gonorrhea.

970 (C) They are subdivided on whether they ferment lactose or not and then further subdivided based on antigenic properties.

971. (D) It is normally endemic.

972. (C) It may even produce macropapular dermatitis.

973. (B) S. typhimurium is the most common of the salmonella causing this.

974. (B) They are particularly good for Rocky Mountain spotted fever and typhus-type infections.

975. (D) Only sulfones are highly effective.

976. (D) Sulfones interfere with nutrition of the causative agent. Too toxic for other uses.

977. (C) Stool mucus is usually rich in the microorganisms.

978. (D) Only D accurately describes an antigen. Some are nonprotein and not all foreign materials produce antibodies.

979. (E) There is no class known as somatophilic.

980. (B) Hypersensitivity to horse serum is quite common

981. (D) Cloudiness or lack of color indicates chemical change.

982. (E) All four are advantages that have contributed to their increased use.

983. (D) It is a viral disease of man found particularly in tropical climates.

984. (D) Agglutination means clumping or aggregation.

985. (A) It is an absolute term.

986. (C) Usually due to subcritical dose of drug agent.

987. (D) Very effective against gram-negative organisms and active at urinary tract pH.

988. (E) Acid-fast bacteria have stored fatty acids, esters, waxes, and mycolic acid.

989. (C) This exotoxin is among the most highly toxic substances known.

990. (D) Viruses and rickettsiae require living tissue, but bacteria will grow on synthetic media.

991. (B) Frequently occur together.

992. (D) The two drugs are almost totally comparable.

993. (A) Direct lethal action on entamoeba histolytica.

994. (E) They are rapid, common, and not temperature-dependent.

995. (A) It is the temperature at which this occurs.

996. (A) This drug is very irritating at infection site.

997. (D) This is Flagyl which is a systemic trichomonacide in both males and females.

998. (C) It is usually given in combination with isoniazid.

999. (A) This is normally found in the mouth along with Borrelia buccalis, but may cause problems under certain conditions.

1000. (A) Based on public health statistics.

1001 (C) Auto means self.

1002. (D) They produce antibodies.

1003. (A) The normal half-life is 14-25 hours. Longest-acting available agent of the class.

1004. (B) It is given once weekly during exposure and for 4-6 weeks after leaving endemic area.

1005. (D) Others will not work, or are too dangerous to use.

1006. (B) This is irreversible discoloration that occurs during the tooth-forming years.

1007. (A) This is a herpes virus.

1008. (D) It can precipitate a severe attack of psoriasis.

1009. (D) This iodine complex is not corrosive, as is free iodine.

1010. (B) This is usually obtained from other persons who previously were infected.

1011. (B) This is the most safe and effective way to immunize.

1012. (E) The purification process removes allergenic materials.

1013. (D) Scarlet fever is caused by alpha hemolytic streptococci.

1014. (B) A glycoprotein which inhibits virus replication.

1015. (A) The average is 18 days.

1016. (B) This is the sole use of spectinomycin.

1017. (B) It is often of value in chronic urinary tract infections.

1018. (D) T. pallidum is a spirochete which causes syphilis.
1019. (A) This is why the term yellow jaundice is often used.
1020. (B) This rickettsia causes epidemic typhus.
1021. (E) Causative organism of venereal disease called chancroid.
1022. (C) The parásite that causes recurrent malaria.

1023. (C) Absorption is delayed.
1024. (D) Synergistic action is seen.
1025. (E) Results in malabsorption of penicllin V.
1026. (B) Increased toxicity is common.
1027. (A) Increases half-life of cetotoxamine.

1028. (A) More easily transmitted from nose due to coughing and sneezing.

1029. (C) May cause weakness of the valves

1030. (E) Most other varieties are heat labile.

1031. (C) It is too toxic for systemic use.

1032. (B) Toxin produced by Clostridia spreads rapidly and has a necrotizing action.

1033. (D) Pyo means pus and derm means skin.

1034. (E) All of these organisms have been implicated.

1035. (A) Speeds up the process markedly.

1036. (C) A number of Shigella species can cause this.

1037. (D) Scars the tubes and causes sterility if untreated.

1038. (D) Difficult to filter, moist methods are unacceptable and others do not give enough penetration.

1039. (C) It is the most potent fungicide.

1040. (D) Candida albicans is the causative fungus.

1041. (E) There is no toxin known as emolosin.

1042. (B) These are highly specific viruses that use the bacteria as hosts.

1043. (A) Weil-Felix is an agglutination reaction with rickettsia, and typhus fever is caused by rickettsiae.

1044. (B) This is a fungus infection and so amphotericin B is the only useful agent listed.

1045. (A) These are proteins formed in response to antigens.

1046. (A) It is particulary useful against herpes simplex.

1047. (B) It is a common type of dermatitis.

1048. (D) Furadantin is particularly effective.

1049. (B) Most of the spotted fevers are rickettsial in origin.

1050. (C) Active ethyl groups attach.

1051. (D) Causes blastomycosis.

1052. (E) The two are synergistic against Pseudomonas.

1053. (B) This produces penicillin G.

1054 (A) C. welchii produces the tissue destruction.

1055 (B) They both belong to the aminoglycoside class.

1056. (C) It is produced by a lichinous form of this bacteria.

1057. (A) The antibodies interact directly with the toxin.

1058. (C) It is effective against all forms of leprosy.

1059. (B) Tolnaftate is a specific antifungal used for athlete's foot and ringworm.

1060. (D) Bubbles appear if there are leaks in HEPA filters.

1061. (C) Particularly good to combat Neisseria, Clostridia and severe staphylococcus infections.

1062. (D) Rheumatic fever is caused by a streptococcus.

1063. (B) Although gallbladder is most common, the urinary tract may be involved.

1064. (A) Applied in topical cream once or twice daily.

1065. (D) Antibodies are depleted rapidly.

1066. (B) These are filters which remove particles from air.

1067. (C) Have a similar spectrum to penicillin G or V.

1068. (A) This is a parasite capable of entering the body through intact skin.

1069. (D) It is a purified protein-derivative multiple-puncture device.

1070. (D) Bacteriostatics inhibit the growth phase.

1071. (C) Massive amount of histamine is produced by foreign protein or antigen.

1072. (D) It is used mainly for thrush and moniliasis.

1073. (B) Most penicillins are produced in this way because it is economical.

1074. (A) It is effective against beef and fish tapeworms.

1075. (B) Need rapid exposure of infected area to remove anaerobic conditions.

1076. (B) They spread to tissues in circulating blood and could not spread by other means.

1077. (D) It is too toxic for routine use.

1078. (D) This is another name for mumps.

1079. (B) C. botulinum is found most commonly in soil, but occasionally in animal feces.

1080. (E) Various species of Proteus can cause all these conditions.

1081. (E) This is the scientific name for common chickenpox.

1082. (B) Nonliving materials such as instruments, needles, etc.

1083. (C) Usually occurs only under a specialized set of conditions which promotes overgrowth.

1084. (A) It acts much faster because of rapid and complete absorption.

1085. (A) This potent sulfonamide is used to prevent sepsis.

1086. (A) It is a mixture of live mumps and rubella virus.

1087. (B) No polymorphic leukocytosis seen.

1088. (B) It has proven to be more effective than other tetracyclines.

1089. (B) Urticaria is the term for the wheals produced by histamine.

1090. (E) All will produce immunity, but the natural way is to contract the disease.

1091. (B) Suby's Solution G is an acidic genitourinary irrigant.

1092. (C) This is the main portal of entry. The virus first multiplies in the tonsils.

1093. (A) This is one definition of vaccination.

1094. (C) Due to improper handling or storage. (Usually poor sealing).

1095. (C) This organism has an affinity for bone.

1096. (A) Autogenous means self-generated.

1097. (B) Volatile halogenated hydrocarbons.

1098. (B) Usually due to seepage of sewage into water supply.

1099. (B) It is a long-acting broad-spectrum antibiotic.

1100. (D) Metronidazole is used to treat entamoeba histolytica.

1101. (B) Triplelennamine is a member of the ethylenediamine class of antihistamines.

1102. (D) Both alcohols and aldehydes are readily oxidized to the corresponding acid.

1103. (C) Gives a brick-red precipitate with reducing sugars.

1104. (D) Intensity is determined by amount of tetrahydrocannibinol present in marijuana.

1105. (B) It is ethylene-diamine-tetraacetic acid and has 4 carboxyl groups.

1106. (C) Marquis reagent is formaldehyde-sulfuric acid which forms a purple complex with the opium alkaloids.

1107. (D) This one identification test for this alkaloid.

1108. (A) It replaces nicotine in tobacco for weaning purposes.

1109. (C) It is chemically $CHCl_3$.

1110. (D) It is a hydrate of the diol aldehyde structure.

1111. (B) It may also be used to detect other metals.

1112. (A) Aspirin hydrolyzes to salicylic acid and acetic acid.

1113. (E) They are R-Mg-X compounds which are used as intermediates in synthesis.

1114. (C) It is based on the fact that different molecular arrangements have different magnetic spin characteristics.

1115. (C) They can accept or donate protons.

1116. (A) They promote water retention in fecal mass.

1117. (C) Reaction is with phenolic hydroxy group.

1118. (D) Has replaced the hydrogen or quinhydrone electroide because of its simplicity and freedom from contamination.

1119. (A) Different densities refract light differently.

1120. (A) Attaches to group and makes it unavailable.

1121. (B) Below 4000 is UV and over 7000 is IR.

1122. (B) Na_2SO_4 is the formula, and substances react in a 2 to 1 ratio.

1123. (D) Formula is $CH_3(CH_2)_{16}COOH$.

1124. (D) Sucrose is a disaccharide made up of a glucose and a fructose molecule.

1125. (E) All of these contain more or less than 16 carbon atoms.

1126. (C) Very long-acting bright color.
1127. (A) All barium salts give this.
1128. (B) Easily masked by other ions and slow to appear.
1129. (D) Some reddish tinge in violet is noticeable.
1130. (E) Very persistent and may mask other ions.

1131. (E) Benzene ring with single hydroxy group.
1132. (D) Common name is chloroform.
1133. (A) Ether USP is $(CH_3 - CH_2)_2$ 0.
1134. (B) Glycerin has OH group on each of three carbon atoms.
1135. (C) Toluene is the monomethyl derivative of benzene.

1136. (C) This salt comes from a weak base and a strong acid. Others are neutral or basic in reaction.

1137. (E) $(1 \times 10^{-7})(1 \times 10^{-7}) = 1 \times 10^{-14}$

1138. (A) All of the ultra-short barbiturates contain S. Longer-acting ones do not.

1139. (B) Insoluble precipitate formed.
1140. (A) Gives a green color.
1141. (A) Gives a red color
1142. (A) Gives a brick-red color.
1143. (D) It is a strong base.

1144. (B) Establishes volume-pressure relationship of gases at constant temperature.
1145. (A) Follows ideal gas law.
1146. (C) Establishes pressure-temperature relationship of constant volumes of gases.

1147. (B) Tendency to offset change.

1148. (B) Sodium hydroxide is strong base and carbonic acid is a weak acid.
1149. (A) OH group on benzene ring is very acidic.
1150. (C) Comes from strong base and strong acid.
1151. (B) Strong base and weak acid source.

1152. (C) It is the acetyl ester of salicylic acid.
1153. (A) It contains the barbituric-acid basic nucleus.
1154. (D) This is one of the tween emulsifiers.
1155. (B) It is a hydrated aldehyde.

1156. (B) Acid is a porton donor by definition in B-L theory.
1157. (E) Base is a proton acceptor in B-L theory.
1158. (A) It is the base formed when HCl gives up a proton.
1159. (C) It is a base formed when H_{4+} gives up a proton.
1160. (D) Definition of molal solution.

1161. (F) Iron is involved in hemoglobin formation.
1162. (E) Gold therapy is a drastic treatment for severe arthritis.
1163. (D) Loss of potassium or low potassium levels cause muscular weakness.
1164. (B) Are converted to nitrites which cause vasodilation.
1165. (C) Treatment with radioactive cobalt is fairly standard.
1166. (A) Magnesium compounds are common adsorbents in antacids.

1167. (C) It is a part of the glucose tolerance factor.

1168. (C) It is a propellant gas.
1169. (B) It is a trihydroxyhydrocarbon.
1170. (A) It is dimethylketone.

1171. (C) Cohesive forces reduce flow.
1172. (B) Used mainly for suspensions.
1173. (D) Measurement of absorbed light at a given wave length.
1174. (A) It is obtained by dividing absolute viscosity by the density.

1175. (E) Can be either reversible or not and is not a chemical reaction.

1176. (C) It is used as a bladder irrigant.
1177. (G) It is vitamin C.
1178. (A) It is a mild antiseptic used in the eye, topically, or vaginally.
1179. (B) It forms a protective layer over burn tissue.
1180. (D) It is used to treat athlete's foot or ringworm.
1181. (E) Another name for this acid is vitamin A.
1182. (F) It is an active ingredient of many tanning preparations.

1183. (D) These are weak forces attracting one molecule to another and are not true chemical bonds.

1184. (D) Leuco means white or colorless.
1185. (C) Depression of freezing point by a known concentration can be used to calculate molecular weight for nonionic molecules.
1186. (B) Usually have a different configuration.
1187. (A) Mixture of d and l optical isomers which do not bend light.
1188. (E) Due to structural shifts and is most common in solutions of carbohydrates.
1189. (F) Due to electrostatic attraction and increases as distance between atoms decreases.
1190. (G) Mirror images are nonsuperimposable.

1191. (A) This group is widely used for general anesthesia because of its lack of flammability.

1192. (D) The hydrolization produces amino acids.

1193. (C) This is used in Ehrlich's test and gives a blue or violet color with various compounds containing indole groups.

1194. (C) All other orders are dependent on concentration of one or more substances present.

1195. (C) This is obtained by dividing molecule weight by hydrogen equivalent.

1196. (B) Iodine is absorbed in direct proportion to the degree of unsaturation.

1197. (B) They also may have substitutions at other positions on the benzene ring.

1198. (D) The base is stronger than the acid from which this salt is derived.

1199. (C) It has a molecular weight of 2. Another radioactive form is tritium (MW 3).

1200. (B) It is used to determine concentration of sugars whose solutions are optically active.

1201. (A) Plasma cholinesterase is the principal detoxifier.

1202. (A) Glyceryl guaicolate is an effective expectorant.

1203. (A) Others do not resemble cages.

1204. (B) These are absorbed better.

1205. (B) The complexation may inactivate many drugs.

1206. (C) Schering trade name for gentamycin.
1207. (A) Upjohn trade name for clindamycin.
1208. (B) Beecham trade name for kanamycin.

1209. (A) This is the sodium salt of an organic acid.
1210. (C) This is an ethyl ester of an organic acid.
1211. (E) It results from removal of HOH from two moles of acid.
1212. (B) Acyl is CO-, and halide is chloride.
1213. (D) Acyl is CO-, and amide is $-COHN_2$.

1214. (D) Lugol's solution is called Stronger Iodine Solution.
1215. (F) One of the active ingredients of Desenex is zinc undecylenate.
1216. (A) Acidulin releases hydrochloric acid in vitro.
1217. (G) Ziradryl contains a zirconium salt used as a protectant.
1218. (H) Robitussin contains the expectorant substance, glyceryl guaiacolate.

1219. (C) Collyrium contains boric acid.
1220. (B) Coricidin contains the antihistamine chlortrimeton.
1221. (E) Pectin is one of the adsorbents in Kaopectate.
1222. (J) Cetamium is the active ingredient.
1223. (I) It contains albamycin combined with tetracycline.

1224. (B) This chemical and its salts coat the stomach.

1225. (D) Both alcohol groups are oxidized completely and form HOOC-COOH, which is oxalic acid.

1226. (A) This blue dye binds selectively with lymphatic protein.

1227. (D) Of the 10 essential amino acids, glutamine is not included.

1228. (E) It is secreted by the pancreas, which is a ductless gland.

1229. (D) Enzymes are biological or chemical catalysts and do not take part in a reaction.

1230. (C) This substance is normally destroyed by MAO.

1231. (C) The bitter taste is detectable at much lower concentration than the others.

1232. (B) At this point, the electrical charge is zero due to complete dissociation of species in equilibrium. The isoelectric point is the pH at which this occurs.

1233 (D) A few amino acids are ketogenic but most are glucogenic.

1234. (C) It is the enzyme that oxidizes monoamines.

1235. (C) It decreases the values in thyroid function test.

1236. (D) Physiological heat of combustion is more than twice that of proteins or carbohydrates.

1237. (D) Combines preferentially to prevent oxygen uptake.

1238. (C) Alkalinization and reduction of hypercalcemia are indicated.

1239. (D) Liver glycogen is converted to glucose.

1240. (B) It is not absorbed to any appreciable extent, because of its low solubility.

1241. (D) Apoenzyme is the prosthetic group portion and not a coenzyme.

1242. (A) Deficiency causes megaloblastic anemias. Folic acid synergizes B_{12}.

1243. (C) It is made up of pantethine and adenosine diphosphate.

1244. (E) Dopa and dopamine are intermediates, but biosynthesis originates with tyrosine.

1245. (A) This is the most important buffer system in the body. Phosphates and protein play smaller roles.

1246. (D) Reduces renal clearance and causes build-up of nitrogen waste in blood.

1247. (A) This range maintains proper electrolyte balance.

1248. (B) This drug gives a similar color reaction, as does mephenesin.

1249. (B) Pepsinogen is a precursor and others are not found in gastric juice.

1250. (B) A certain minimum daily protein uptake is necessary to maintain balance.

1251. (A) This in turn slows down protein degradation to uric acid.

1252. (B) This is involved only in the citrate cycle.

1253. (C) The glycogen-glucose equilibrium controls needs of body for energy.

1254. (D) Ferrous porphyrin is the hemo portion of hemoglobin.

1255. (D) Contracts gallbladder and evacuates bile.

1256. (D) Lower or higher values produce hypoglycemia or hyperglycemia.

1257. (D) This is a drug interaction that can delay or prevent clotting.

1258. (E) All are necessary for the cells.

1259. (E) This is a reducing substance and the reaction is based on reduction.

1260. (B) It is a disaccharide formed only in the mammary glands.

1261. (D) Mitochondria are rich in these enzymes.

1262. (C) Glycogen is converted to d-glucose.

1263. (C) This dye stains the mitochondria selectively.

1264. (A) It detects occult blood in urine, stool, or gastric contents.

1265. (E) PBI stands for proetin-bound iodine and iodides elevate the value.

1266. (C) Sulfonamides are substituted paraaminobenzoic acids and serve as competitive inhibitors.

1267. (C) Vitamin A aldehydes are components of visual purple.

1268. (C) It is the principal progestational substance in corpus luteum.

1269. (A) It is a biotransformation.

1270. (C) Others are relatively heat stable.

1271. (C) Forms complex between calcium and citrate ions.

1272. (A) Penicillins and cromolyn have no effect.

1273. (C) Extrinsic source of pancreatin aids digestion.

1274. (A) Lipids and albuminoids are not usually present.

1275. (C) May also be used to treat overdoses of warfarin.

1276. (A) Charge is positive below isoelectric point.

1277. (E) It interferes with urine tests for RBC or hemoglobin.

1278. (B) It is an albuminoid scleroprotein.

1279. (D) Unnecessary if there is high tryptophan content in diet.

1280. (C) Mediates prothrombin formation and aids clotting.

1281. (E) It provides the energy for contraction.

1282. (B) Have no effect on sperm or egg fertilization and do not prevent menses.

1283. (E) Oxidation occurs entirely through coenzyme A intermediates.

1284. (C) Classic drug interaction.

1285. (D) Used only in vitro.

1286. (B) It is similar to histamine but less toxic.

1287. (E) Both affect growth and development of the gonads.

1288. (E) Exact meahanism is not known.

1289. (D) Parathyroid gland is the principal regulator of calcium metabolism.

1290. (E) Range is 90-140 days. Determined by tagging with radioactive tracers.

1291. (D) Converted to vitamin A in the liver.

1292. (A) This is caused by overproduction of purines.

1293. (C) Formed in mast cells of the liver of mammals.

1294. (D) Found in the thyroid glands. It has manv reactive tyrosyl residues.

1295. (D) It fluoresces at the same wave length as catecholamines.

1296. (E) Little iron is eliminated because of the number of storage sites.

1297. (D) Due to oversecretion of pituitary hormones.

1298. (D) It is dependent on pressure of chorionic gonadotropin.

1299. (A) Enzyme systems favor this route.

1300. (B) Has no effect on the other three.

1301. (D) Based on USPHS figures.

1302. (B) B complex and C are mainly water soluble.

1303. (A) Fick's law deals with concentration gradients in passive diffusion.

1304. (C) When extrinsic source is given, intrinsic source compensates.

1305. (C) Body does compensate, but not entirely.

1306. (E) They are precursors of proteolytic enzymes.

1307. (A) Stored until needed for the eye.

1308. (A) Done by hydroxylation and loss of formaldehyde group and later goes to biliverdin and then to bilirubin.

1309. (E) All of these steps are seen.

1310. (C) This is the heme portion.

1311. (C) Aminoacetic acid is required to form globin portion.

1312. (B) Man and apes do not have the appropriate enzyme catalysts.

1313. (C) It acts as an acetylcholine agonist in smooth muscle and the brain.

1314. (E) The prinicpal end product is urea.

1315. (E) It is very similar to thyrotropin releasing hormone.

1316. (D) Vitamin E is preferentially oxidized.

1317. (C) This is the chief function of DNA.

1318. (B) It is a highly alkaline organic amine.

1319. (D) It breaks down starch or other carbohydrates.

1320. (D) Deficiency results in retardation of growth.

1321. (C) ATP is the source of the high energy needed.

1322. (C) Cyanide inactivates this respiratory enzyme.

1323. (B) Debilitated patients show vitamin deficiencies.

1324. (D) Must combine with ferrous because of valence and must be reversible to release oxygen to tissues.

1325. (E) Levels of over 7.5 mg% usually produce severe symptoms.

1326. (B) Acts like a reducing sugar with tests using Benedict's or similar reagents.

1327. (A) Rhodopsin (visual purple) is transformed reversibly by conversion of light to nerve impulses.

1328. (D) They are precursors of this vitamin that is involved in eye functions.

1329. (C) Stimulation of these enzymes may decrease blood levels and efficacy of other drugs given concurrently.

1330. (D) Both contain the basic cyclopentano-perhydrophenanthrene group.

1331. (D) Cholesterol is a lipid and calciferol, tocopherol and biotin are other vitamins.

1332. (B) Glucuronides are common metabolites of drugs containing these groups.

1333. (B) Skin is made up of about 75% collagen.

1334. (A) It is strictly a concentration gradient that establishes equilibrium.

1335. (C) Ionization is depressed at the acid pH of the stomach.

1336. (E) Ribose or desoxyribose is the carbohydrate portion.

1337. (E) Also synthesizes some proteins and fats.

1338. (D) This is the first step in inactivation of these compounds.

1339. (D) They all are 20-carbon-atom fatty acids.

1340. (D) These act as bridges between systems.

1341. (A) Lactic acid is the product of carbohydrate hydrolysis.

1342. (C) Both are dinucleotides made up of nicotinamide and adenine.

1343. (D) Magnesium is necessary for normal muscle contraction and nerve conduction.

1344. (D) It is currently reported that over 90% of patients receiving L-Dopa experience some side effects.

1345. (B) This is also called the citrate cycle. End-products are CO_2 and water.

1346. (A) Might have some if solubility is exceeded, but other factors have much more effect.

1347. (D) Suppresses release of intrinsic insulin.

1348. (D) This is a better way of measuring because it lessens effect of peaks and valleys.

1349. (D) It is necessary for development of taste buds.

1350. (A) Although they are lipid-like, their actions closely resemble that of hormones.

1351. (A) Due to ketoacidosis.

1352. (C) It triggers this center to increase respiration to produce exchange.

1353. (C) It inhibits the motility of the stomach.

1354. (A) It triggers release of O_2 to maintain balance.

1355. (E) Caused by formation of metabolic acids in body or ingestion of metabolic acids or loss of bicarbonate.

1356. (C) This is the record of atrial depolarization.

1357. (A) It is a record of the resistance encountered.

1358. (A) It also releases other thromboplastic factors.

1359. (C) Anuria is complete stoppage of urine flow. Poly uria is increased flow and the other two do not deal with amount of urine.

1360. (E) It is a bone problem of the legs seen in rapidly growing youngsters.

1361. (A) This is the pacemaker of the heart.

1362. (C) They are mediated by acetylcholine.

1363. (A) This narrows the arteries and limits oxygen supply.

1364. (D) All of the vital centers are located here.

1365. (A) It stimulates sodium transport by the tubule.

1366. (B) Successive contractions run together and are indistinguishable.

1367. (E) This varies from one individual to another and is only a rough estimate.

1368. (D) It usually results from impairment or damage of enzyme systems.

1369. (E) Elasticity is closely tied to peripheral resistance.

1370. (A) Up to 50 parallel capillaries encased in Bowman's capsule, in which fluid collects.

1371. (D) It is the area between the proximal and distal tubules.

1372. (A) Usually is correctable by speech therapy.

1373. (A) Has diuretic effect and causes muscle weakness.

1374. (A) These are mobile histiocytes found in nervous tissue.

1375. (B) The key word is ***organized.***

1376. (B) It is excellent because it passes the glomerular membrane easily and is not reabsorbed.

1377. (D) The hypothalamus is also involved.

1378. (D) This hormone can alter the rate of water excretion by a factor of up to 45.

1379. (B) They are autonomic ganglia.

1380. (A) This is the increase above normal and is usually more than 300%.

1381 (C) It is related to clearance of paraaminohippurates. Radioiodine may also be used.

1382. (E) Release hormones into extracellular fluid for circulation.

1383. (B) Epinephrine and norepinephrine are released in the sympathetic system and the two enzymes are not mediators.

1384. (D) This is its chief function.

1385. (E) They are caused by loss of sodium through sweating.

1386. (C) It is 16 g for men and 14 g for women on the average.

1387. (A) The normal range is usually 42–45%.

1388. (A) These are types of white blood cells.

1389. (D) The stomach empties directly into the duodenum. The ileum and jejunum are lower.

1390. (A) Others may change basic color, however.

1391. (B) Secreted by adrenal medulla.
1392. (A) Triggered by pregnancy.
1393. (C) Secreted by isles of Langerhans in pancreas.
1394. (E) Involved with iodine metabolism.
1395. (D) Derives its name from the stomach.
1396. (A) Male sex hormone secreted and regulated by this gland.
1397. (A) This is the adrenocorticotrophic hormone, but it is secreted by the master gland.

1398. (C) Usually caused by pulmonary or vascular disease which produces severe congestion at right ventricle of heart.

1399. (C) Failure to equalize may cause pain and require myringotomy.

1400. (B) All of the others stimulate secretion.

1401. (B) Gray matter integrates reflexes and white matter conducts them.

1402. (D) It is involved in blood clotting but originates in the liver.

1403. (A) Tissues must be kept clean and debrided.

1404. (B) This is the postganglionic mediator.

1405. (B) The term for dilation of the pupil is mydriasis.

1406. (C) About 46% of all persons have this type. Type A is the next most common.

1407. (C) It is caused by chronic adrenocortical insufficiency.

1408. (B) Hypothalmic thermostat conserves heat, and then pyrogens from microorganisms cause it to increase heat production.

1409. (A) It is an elastic-like response.

1410. (B) It is stimulated to release O_2.

1411. (F) Balance center is located in labyrinth.
1412. (H) Rods are responsible for night vision.
1413. (D) It is the connecting pathway during pregnancy.
1414. (A) Combines reversibly with oxygen.
1415. (B) Primary phagocytes of the body.
1416. (C) Regulates blood pressure.
1417. (E) Stimulation will slow the heart.
1418. (G) Transmits electrical impulse in the heart.

1419. (D) They transmit impulse to entire heart.

1420. (C) The impulse arises at this node.

1421. (B) Overstimulation may produce convulsions.

1422. (D) Others are not energy sources.

1423. (D) Usually associated with disease of lungs or bronchi.

1424. (D) It involves chronic enlargement of lymph nodes.

1425. (C) Used for clearance test.

1426. (C) It is an in vitro test for antibiotics.

1427. (D) Phagocytize particles and foreign proteins.

1428. (E) Most commonly found in the signoid colon after age 40.

1429. (C) Made up of second order neurons.

1430. (D) Effects are massive and usually irreversible.

1431. (A) Also means person is far-sighted.

1432. (D) There is marked loss of function.

1433. (D) These are needed to dissolve fatty substances.

1434. (B) Usually caused by Histoplasma capsulatum, a soil fungus.

1435. (B) AV valves of this pump produce sound.

1436. (B) Found in stomach area.

1437. (D) Stimulates respiratory center directly.

1438. (C) Principal intrinsic ion.

1439. (A) Interstices are rich in sodium.

1440. (C) They are powerful protein precipitants and create massive imbalance.

1441. (C) From the Greek *xeros* meaning dry and *stoma* meaning mouth.

1442. (C) Type of anemia caused by excessive number of red blood cells.

1443. (B) These are vital reflex centers.

1444. (C) It is converted to bicarbonate.

1445. (C) Slowing of the heart as if for compensation.

1446. (C) This triggers expulsion of bile.

1447. (B) Other components do not contribute to pH.

1448. (C) It is the end-product of degradation.

1449. (B) These are the ducts to the bladder.

1450. (B) It concentrates bile tenfold.

1451. (C) Used as plasma expanders.

1452. (B) Foot should not be immersed in any liquid.

1453. (C) Expansion of diameter slows flow proportionately.

1454. (D) Also known as ulcerating gingivitis or trench mouth.

1455. (D) Also called esophagism.

1456. (A) It is a sympathomimetic.
1457. (B) Opium alkaloids constrict pupil to pinpoint size.
1458. (B) It is a potent diuretic.
1459. (B) There is less volume excreted.
1460. (B) It is an anticholinergic used to dry secretions
1461. (A) They are emulsifiers and aid in absorption.
1462. (A) They are mobilized to help with phagocytosis.
1463. (A) They prevent MAO from destroying serotonin.
1464. (B) Slows peristalsis and causes constipation.
1465. (C) Affects only RBC.

1466. (C) This is the innervative mechanism.

1467. (C) Each unit of blood contains about 250 mg of iron.

1468. (D) It is ulcerative colitis.

1469. (C) Subject to rupture.

1470. (D) They constitute 60% of all white blood cells.

1471. (D) Calcium is needed to maintain normal state.

1472. (C) This derivative is formed there.

1473. (A) It is a jerking movement of the eyes.

1474. (D) It is necessary to trigger or stop secretion.

1475. (D) Injury and toxic chemicals also cause this, but septicemia is a common cause.

1476. (C) It is a glucocorticoid.

1477. (A) These are the immunoglobulins.

1478. (D) The lens focuses the images on the retina.

14. (C) It is a thin membrane interspersed between the ural cavity and the capillaries.

1480. (C) Connects ganglia to the brain by this.

1481. (A) It is actually about 15/40 on the average.

1482. (A) Usually involves fibrosis and scarring.

1483. (C) More usual to use PQ interval, but PR interval is quite close in value.

1484. (A) These have great surface area which aids in absorption.

1485. (D) Some antacids may stimulate increase in rate and acidity of gastric secretions.

1486. (A) There is loss of total function and tissue death.

1487. (B) *Sphygmo* is the Greek for pulse and *meter* denotes measure.

1488. (B) The 46 are arranged in 23 pairs.

1489. (D) May be due to a genetic error in the mitotic control system.

1490. (A) Hippurates measure tubular function only.
1491. (C) Combination needed to measure both.
1492. (B) Insulin measures glomerular filtration.

1493. (A) Greek word *sternos* means chest.

1494. (D) Derived from Greek *dys* meaning bad and *pnoe* meaning breathing.

1495. (E) Cyst means bladder and its ending means inflammation.

1496. (C) Varies somewhat with sex, weight and other factors.

1497. (C) Abnormal shape can cause vascular occlusions.

1498. (A) Both mean a fear of heights.

1499. (E) Muscle that flexes thigh and leg.

1500. (C) Glucagon is a metabolic counterweight to insulin.

BIBLIOGRAPHY

Current Medical Diagnosis and Treatment, Krupp, M. and Chatton, M., Lange, Los Altos, CA: 1975.

Medical Pharmacology, Goth, A., 5th Edition, C.V. Mosby, St. Louis: 1976.

National Formulary, American Pharmaceutical Association, 14th Edition, Mack, Easton, PA: 1975.

Pharmacologic Basis of Therapeutics, Goodman, L. and Gilman, A. (Ed.), 5th Edition, MacMillan, NY: 1975.

Pharmacology and Drug Therapy in Nursing, Rodman, Morton J. and Smith, Dorothy W. (Ed.), J.B. Lippincott, NY: 1968.

Prescription Pharmacy, Sprowls, J, 2nd Edition, J.B. Lippincott, Philadelphia: 1970.

Remington's Pharmaceutical Sciences, Osol, A. et al., 15th Edition, Mack, Easton, PA: 1975.

Review of Medical Pharmacology, Meyers, F., Jawetz, E., and Goldfein, A., 6th Edition, Lange, Los Altos, CA: 1978.

United States Pharmacopoeial Convention, 19th Edition, Mack, Easton, PA: 1975.